ABC OF HYPERTENSION

Th:

ABC OF HYPERTENSION

THIRD EDITION

EOIN O'BRIEN
Professor of Cardiovascular Medicine, Blood Pressure Unit
Beaumont Hospital, Dublin

D GARETH BEEVERS
Professor of Medicine
City Hospital, Birmingham

HOWARD J MARSHALL
Research Fellow
Queen Elizabeth Hospital, Birmingham

First published in 1981
by the BMJ Publishing Group, BMA House, Tavistock Square,
London WC1H 9JR

First edition 1981
Fifth impression 1985
Second edition 1987
Second impression 1988
Third impression 1988
Fourth impression 1988
Fifth impression 1989
Third edition 1995

British Library Cataloguing in Publication Data

A catalogue record for this book is available from the
British Library

ISBN 0-7279-0769-7

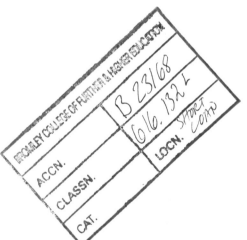

Typeset by Apek Typesetters Ltd, Nailsea, Bristol
Printed in Great Britain by Eyre & Spottiswoode, Margate

Contents

PREFACE TO THE THIRD EDITION

The *ABC of Hypertension*, which first appeared in the *BMJ* in 1980, was published in book form soon after and an extensively revised second edition was produced in 1987. These two earlier editions now make interesting reading as they demonstrate the radical changes that have taken place over the past 15 years in clinical "hypertensionology," as well as in graphic design. This new third edition again is a total and comprehensive re-working of the whole topic of hypertension and its management. The format of short, clear well illustrated chapters has, however, been retained as it proved so popular with readers. Some of the statements we have made may seem a little dogmatic or didactic, but they are based on our interpretation of the published evidence and the opinions of our colleagues.

As in the earlier editions considerable emphasis has been given to the measurement of blood pressure. Diagnostic, therapeutic, and prognostic decisions are based, after all, on the level of blood pressure determined by a technique which has many shortcomings. This realisation has motivated much research over the past decade into devising and assessing new methods of measurement, a trend that has been facilitated by the application of advances in technology. The most notable development has been the technique of 24-hour ambulatory blood pressure measurement. With recognition of the phenomenon of "white coat hypertension" it has become evident that future attention will be directed more to the behaviour of blood pressure over time and under differing circumstances rather than basing decisions, as hitherto, on a limited number of measurements, often obtained under stressful circumstances.

Probably the two main advances in the management of hypertension since 1987 are the increasing awareness of the importance of hypertension in elderly people, including isolated systolic hypertension, and the steadily expanding role of the angiotensin converting enzyme (ACE) inhibitors. Both these trends need to be seen from the perspective of the management of the whole patient and not just of his or her blood pressure. The rigid stepped care approach of the 1981 edition has been replaced by a more flexible tailored-care, taking into account concommittant risk factors or diseases, previous end-organ damage, and side effects of drugs. One can at this stage only speculate whether the advent of the angiotensin receptor antagonists will have a similar impact as the ACE inhibitors. With five (and soon six) different classes of anti-hypertensive drugs available the clinician now has the freedom to chose the optimum drug for the patient and should actively elicit side-effects of the drugs or specifically avoid them in high risk groups.

Antihypertensive drug therapy prevents strokes and heart attacks and the main challenge now is to ensure that this validated form of health care is made available to all who need it. The practicalities of this are mainly the concern of general practitioners, for whom this third edition is written. We hope that readers will find it useful.

D G Beevers
E O'Brien
H J Marshall
March 1995

PART I

BLOOD PRESSURE MEASUREMENT

E O'BRIEN

GENERAL PRINCIPLES OF BLOOD PRESSURE MEASUREMENT

SPHYGMOMANOMETERS

Historical milestones in blood pressure measurement

- 1733: the Reverend Stephen Hales performed his famous experiment demonstrating that blood rose to a height of 8 feet 3 inches in a glass tube placed in the artery of a horse
- 1828: blood pressure in animals measured directly with a mercury sphygmomanometer by Jean-Leonard Marie Poiseuille
- 1847: introduction of the kymograph by Carl Ludwig
- 1855: introduction of the sphygmograph by Karl Vierordt
- 1850–90: development of sphygmographs by Marey, Mahomed, and Dudgeon
- 1880: introduction of the "sphygmomanometer" of von Basch
- 1880–90: modifications to von Basch sphygmomanometer by Potain, Hill, and Barnard
- 1896: Scipione Riva-Rocci introduced an arm-occluding mercury sphygmomanometer which could record systolic blood pressure accurately in clinical conditions
- 1897: Hill and Barnard developed an arm-occluding aneroid sphygmomanometer
- 1904: Theodore Janeway drew attention to the variability of blood pressure and the striking response to stresses such as surgery, tobacco, and anxiety
- 1905: the Russian surgeon, Nicolai Sergeivich Korotkov, presented the technique of auscultatory measurement of systolic and diastolic blood pressure to the Imperial Military Academy in St Petersburg
- 1940: Ayman and Goldshine showed that blood pressure measured at home was lower than in the clinic
- 1944: Smirk assessed blood pressure behaviour in the individual by measuring basal blood pressure
- 1964: George Pickering showed for the first time the constant nature of and profound fall in blood pressure recorded during sleep.
- 1964: Hinman described the first truly portable ambulatory system for the non-invasive measurement of blood pressure — the Remler M-2000

Sphygmomanometry has evolved over nearly three centuries and as we approach the end of the twentieth century the advent of automated devices heralds a change of direction in blood pressure measurement.

Although conventional sphygmomanometry using the technique introduced by Riva-Rocci in 1896 and modified by Korotkov in 1905 has served us well for the past 100 years, a new era has dawned.

We may now anticipate the demise of the conventional method of blood pressure measurement using the mercury sphygmomanometer after nearly a century of use in clinical practice, although it may be retained as a gold standard in validation research. The reasons for this are twofold. First, the pressure from environmentalists to ban mercury as a toxic substance is likely to be persuasive, as indeed it has been in Scandinavian countries and to a great extent in

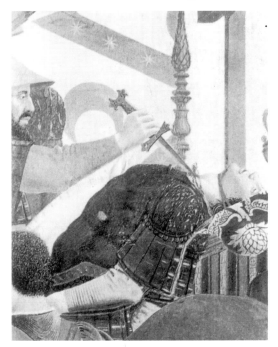

The Legend of the True Cross. Detail from *The battle between Heraclius and Chosroes* by Piero della Francesca (1415/20–92). Arezzo. Church of S. Francesco. (From Murray and de Vecchi, 1987, with permission). The concept of blood pressure was clearly recognised by the artist.

Nicolai Sergeivich Korotkov. (From Segall, 1981)

3

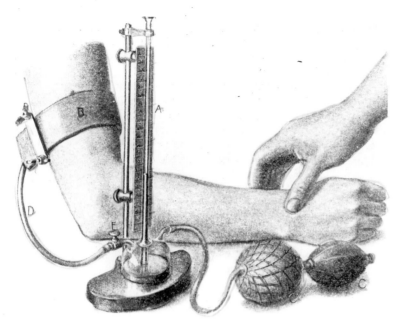

Riva-Rocci sphygmomanometer. (From Janeway, 1904, p.79)

the United States of America. But even if a non-toxic equivalent was found for mercury, the reality is that accurate automated devices will soon replace the conventional technique which is flawed by inaccuracy from observer prejudice. In fact the development of computer assisted techniques for blood pressure measurement opens boundless possibilities with the likelihood that ambulatory measurement will become inexpensive. It is accurate and, when shown to be superior to conventional measurement in predicting prognosis, it will become indispensable in the assessment of the hypertensive patient.

The inadequacy of bladder size is a major cause of inaccuracy for all techniques of blood pressure measurement dependent on cuff occlusion, and it is not unreasonable to anticipate the development of a cuff that is adjustable for all arms in the near future.

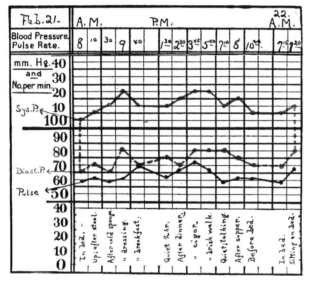

Diurnal blood pressure chart of a healthy man.
(From Janeway, 1904, p.114)

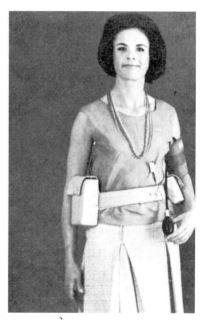

The Remler ambulatory blood pressure recorder.
(From Kain et al, 1964, with permission)

General principles of blood pressure measurement

Blood pressure measurement is one of the few scientific measurements undertaken by doctors in the course of clinical assessment and it occupies more of nurses' time, on the wards, in the accident and emergency department, and in the outpatient departments, than any other measurement. The situation is similar in family practice. The consequences of decisions arising from the measurement of blood pressure may be crucial to patient management in the short term and, perhaps more importantly, the level of blood pressure recorded may influence the quality of life for the remainder of a patient's life. Whatever the circumstances or the device used for measuring blood

Important factors affecting measurement

- Being aware of the inherent variability of blood pressure
- The defence reaction
- The limitations of the device being used
- The accuracy of the device
- Blood pressure is not as easily measured in some groups, such as elderly people

pressure, there are certain principles that must be recognised in the performance and interpretation of blood pressure, if measurement is to be used correctly in the assessment of the overall cardiovascular status of an individual.

Most devices depend on occlusion of an artery of an extremity with an occluding cuff to measure blood pressure either by oscillometry or by detection of Korotkov sounds, although other techniques may be used, such as pulse waveform analysis. The occluding cuff and bladder can influence the accuracy of blood pressure measurement regardless of the technique employed for detecting blood pressure.

The cuff and bladder

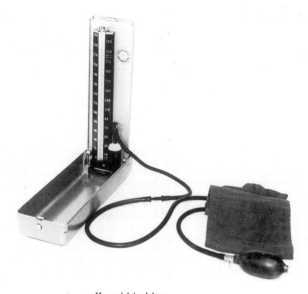

Sphygmomanometer cuff and bladder

The cuff is an inelastic cloth that encircles the arm and encloses the inflatable rubber bladder. It is secured round the arm, most commonly by means of Velcro on the adjoining surfaces of the cuff, occasionally by wrapping a tapering end into the encircling cuff, and rarely by hooks.

Tapering cuffs should be long enough to encircle the arm several times: the full length should extend beyond the end of the inflatable bladder for 25 cm and then should gradually taper for a further 60 cm. Velcro surfaces must be effective, and when they lose their grip the cuff should be discarded. It should be possible to remove the bladder from the cuff so that the cuff can be washed from time to time.

Mismatching of bladder and arm

Bladder too small *Undercuffing*	Overestimation of BP Range of error: 3·2/2·4– 12/8 mm Hg, as much as 30 mm Hg in obesity
Bladder too large *Overcuffing*	Underestimation of BP Range of error: 10– 30 mm Hg

Undercuffing more common than *overcuffing*

Miscuffing

There is no agreement about the optimal bladder dimensions for a particular arm circumference. The use of cuffs containing inappropriately sized bladders is a serious source of error which must inevitably lead to incorrect diagnosis. There is unequivocal evidence that either too narrow or too short a bladder will cause overestimation of blood pressure and equivocal evidence that too wide or too long a bladder may cause underestimation of blood pressure. In clinical practice a bladder that is too short or too narrow will result in overdiagnosis of hypertension, and one that is too long or too wide may cause the condition to be underdiagnosed. The magnitude of the error resulting from mismatch of the bladder to arm size will obviously vary according to the degree of mismatching.

Arm circumference

Overestimation of blood pressure with too small a bladder ranges from 14% to 37%. In one study 300 000 adults in England and Wales might have been treated unnecessarily as a result of overestimation of blood pressure resulting from the use of too small a bladder. If the conservative Swedish estimate of £40 (US$26) as being the annual cost of treating a patient with hypertension is applied to these figures an unnecessary expenditure of £12 million (US$8 million) per annum is incurred.

Underestimation resulting from the use of too large a bladder is a smaller problem, with one study showing that 30% of hypertensive subjects were misdiagnosed as normotensive because the bladder was

Sphygmomanometers

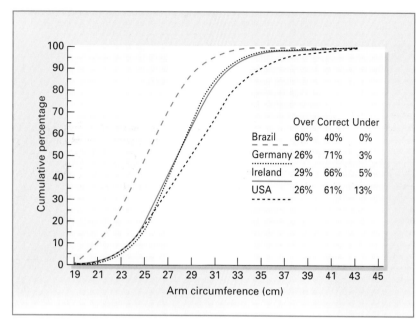

	Over	Correct	Under
Brazil	60%	40%	0%
Germany	26%	71%	3%
Ireland	29%	66%	5%
USA	26%	61%	13%

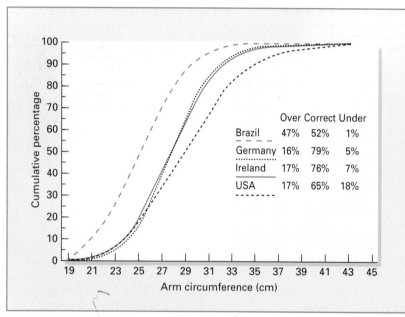

	Over	Correct	Under
Brazil	47%	52%	1%
Germany	16%	79%	5%
Ireland	17%	76%	7%
USA	17%	65%	18%

The effect of altering bladder length in different populations with varying arm circumferences: correct cuffing using 27 cm bladder (top) and 26 cm bladder (bottom). From these plots it is evident that as little as 1 cm in bladder length influences the percentage of the population that is correctly cuffed or under or overcuffed.

too large. It has been suggested that use of a bladder suitable for the arms of people in the Western World may have led to underestimation of the prevalence of hypertension in a Brazilian population.

In deciding what constitutes the optimum cuff for clinical sphygmomanometry, the first step is to determine the dimensions of the arms of different populations.

The American Heart Association recommends that the width of the inflatable bladder should be 12–14 cm, or 40% of the circumference of the midpoint of the arm (with narrower bladders for children and wider ones for obese subjects), and that the length should be 80% of the arm circumference, with adult lengths of 17, 24, 32, and 42 cm (thigh) bladder lengths being recommended. These recommendations necessitate the provision of five cuffs in the wards, outpatient, and accident and emergency departments of general hospitals, and three in children's hospitals, with family practitioners being required to stock all eight cuffs. This is clearly not feasible in practice. The British Hypertension Society and the British Standards Institute (BHS/BSI) have recommended a cuff containing a bladder 12 x 35 cm on the basis that this will give accurate blood pressure measurements in most adults, that is, those with arm circumferences measuring 35–42 cm, but in subjects with arm circumferences below 35 cm blood pressure will be underestimated. It might be argued that because so many factors — the alarm reaction, white coat hypertension, and regression to the mean, for example — mitigate to give erroneously high blood pressure measurements a tendency to underestimate may be no bad thing. In subjects with arm circumferences over 42 cm, blood pressure will be overestimated and this may have more serious consequences in terms of misdiagnosis.

The arm circumference of 1300 Irish men and women ranging in age from 17 to 80 years was measured. Mean arm circumference was 30·2 cm (±4 cm). A review of the literature from other European countries shows that an arm circumference of 30 cm is about average. Applying the American Heart Association criterion that a bladder should be long enough to encircle at least 80% of the arm, a bladder measuring 26 × 12 cm would correctly cuff 79% of arms in this population, and incorrectly cuff 21% of arms — 10% from undercuffing and 11% from overcuffing. Using the BHS/BSI recommended bladder, only 6% of arms would be correctly cuffed with 94% being overcuffed and none being undercuffed. The error introduced by this degree of overcuffing is not known, although these findings suggest that the optimum bladder dimensions should be recommended according to the arm circumference of the population for which the recommendation applies, and that current recommendations for bladder length may be excessive, resulting in overcuffing in most of the population. It would seem appropriate, therefore, to have three cuffs available that contain bladders with the dimensions shown in the box.

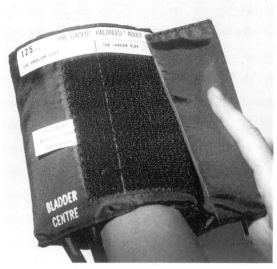

Markings on the cuff

Markers on cuffs

Some cuffs carry an imprint of a "range" on the interior border of the cuff, others an indelible marker on the interior surface of the cuff at a distance 32 cm from the left border in the standard cuff and 42 cm from the left border in the large adult cuff, as a "built in" measurement of arm circumference which allows recognition of miscuffing.

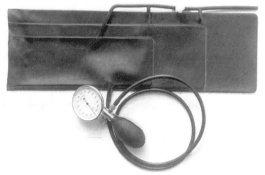

The TriCuff

Combination cuffs

A cuff containing three inflatable bladders of varying dimensions has been designed for use in subjects with arm circumferences ranging from 24 to 42 cm, but the extra rigidity in the cuff may introduce error and the cuff has not yet been fully evaluated.

Inflation–deflation system

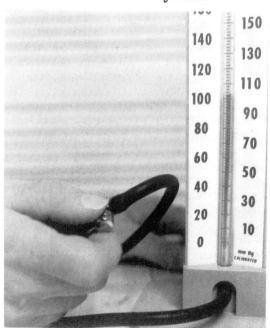

Inflation/deflation mechanism and rubber tubing

The inflation–deflation system consists of an inflating and deflating mechanism connected by rubber tubing to an occluding bladder. Automated devices, of which there are many varieties, operate on the principle that, once the device has been activated, it inflates automatically to a programmed cuff pressure and then deflates automatically, sensing the blood pressure most commonly with a microphone although increasingly by oscillometry and ultrasonography. The recorded pressure may then be stored and/or displayed on a screen or printed.

The standard mercury and aneroid sphygmomanometers used in clinical practice are operated manually; inflation is effected by means of a bulb compressed by hand and deflation by means of a release valve which is also controlled by hand. The pump and control valve are connected to the inflatable bladder and thence to the sphygmomanometer by rubber tubing.

Rubber tubing

Leaks resulting from cracked or perished rubber make accurate measurement of blood pressure difficult because the fall in mercury cannot be controlled. The rubber should be in a good condition and free from leaks. The minimum length of tubing between the cuff and the manometer should be 70 cm and between the inflation source and the cuff 30 cm. Connections should be air tight and easily disconnected.

Standards for blood pressure measuring devices

The British Hypertension Society protocol for the evaluation of blood pressure measuring devices

Eoin O'Brien, James Petrie, William Littler, Michael de Swiet, Paul L Padfield, Douglas G Altman, Martin Bland, Andrew Coats, and Neil Atkins
Journal of Hypertension 1993, **11** (suppl 2):S43–62

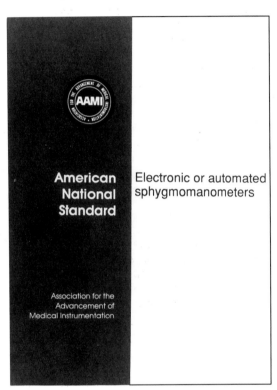

American National Standard

Electronic or automated sphygmomanometers

Association for the Advancement of Medical Instrumentation

There are two published standards for the evaluation of devices for measuring blood pressure: the American Association for the Advancement of Medical Instrumentation (AAMI) standard, which is accepted by the Food and Drug Administration as the national standard in the USA, and the more comprehensive protocol of the British Hypertension Society (BHS).

Manufacturers are not at present obliged to guarantee the accuracy of their product, although most reputable manufacturers welcome the opportunity of having their devices evaluated independently, according to a generally accepted protocol. The European Community has established a working party to draw up a standard for all devices measuring blood pressure and a directive will be issued in 1995 that will be legally binding on all member states.

Acknowledgments

Janeway TC. *The clinical study of blood-pressure.* D. Appleton & Co., New York, London, 1904:79

Kain HK, Hinman AT, Sokolow M. Arterial blood pressure measurements with a portable recorder in hypertensive patients. I. Variability and correlation with "casual" pressures. *Circulation* 1964;**30**: 882–92.

Murray P, de Vecchi P. *The complete paintings of Piero della Francesca.* Penguin Classics of World Art, Penguin Books, Middlesex, 1987.

Segall HN. Discussion of Dr. de Moulin's presentation on the history of blood pressure measurement. *Second Eithoven meeting on past and present cardiology: blood pressure measurement and systemic hypertension.* Eds, A.C. Arntzenius, A.J. Dunning, H.A. Snellen. Medical World Press, Breda, The Netherlands, 1981;35.

Working Party of EC. *Non-invasive sphygmomanometers.* CEN/TC 205/WG 10.

Further reading

O'Brien E, Fitzgerald D. The history of indirect blood pressure measurement. In: Birkenhager WH, Reid JL, series eds. *Handbook of hypertension.* Vol. 14. O'Brien E, O'Malley K, eds. *Blood pressure measurement.* Amsterdam: Elsevier, 1991:1–54.

O'Brien E. Blood pressurement measurement. In: JD Swales, ed. *Textbook of hypertension.* Oxford: Blackwell Scientific Publications, 1994:989–1008.

O'Brien E, O'Malley K. Clinical blood pressure measurement. In: Birkenhager WH, Reid JL, series eds. *Handbook of hypertension.* Vol. 15. Robertson JIS, ed. *Clinical hypertension.* Amsterdam: Elsevier, 1992:14–50.

Petrie JC, O'Brien ET, Littler WA, de Swiet M. Recommendations on blood pressure measurement. British Hypertension Society. *BMJ* 1986;**293**:611–5.

Petrie JC, O'Brien ET, Littler WA, de Swiet M, Dillon MJ, Padfield PL. *Recommendations on blood pressure measurements.* 2nd ed. London: BMJ Publishing Group, 1990.

Maxwell MH, Waks AU, Schroth PC, Karam M, Dornfeld LP. Error in blood-pressure measurement due to incorrect cuff size in obese patients. *Lancet* 1982;**ii**:33–6.

Croft PR, Cruikshank JK. Blood pressure measurement in adults: large cuffs for all? *J Epidemiol Commun Health* 1990;**44**:170–3.

O'Brien E, Petrie J, Littler WA, de Swiet M, Padfield PL, Altman D, Bland M, Coats A, Atkins N. An outline of the British Hypertension Society Protocol for the evaluation of blood pressure measuring devices. *J Hypertens* 1993;**11**:677–9.

O'Brien E, Petrie J, Littler WA, de Swiet M, Padfield PL, Altman D, Bland M, Coats A, Atkins N. The British Hypertension Society Protocol for the evaluation of blood pressure measuring devices. *J Hypertens* 1993;**11**(suppl 2):S43–63.

FACTORS AFFECTING BLOOD PRESSURE

Variability of blood pressure

Various factors affecting blood pressure
• Respiration
• Emotion
• Exercise
• Meals
• Tobacco
• Alcohol
• Temperature
• Bladder distension
• Pain

The observer must be aware of the considerable variability that may occur in blood pressure from moment to moment from various factors. These include emotion, exercise, respiration, meals, tobacco, alcohol, temperature, pain, and bladder distension.

Blood pressure is also influenced by age, race, and circadian variation. It is usually at its lowest during sleep. It is not always possible to modify so many factors but we can minimise their effect by taking them into account in reaching a decision about the relevance or otherwise of a particular blood pressure measurement.

In so far as is practical, the patient should be relaxed in a quiet room at a comfortable temperature, and a short period of rest should precede the measurement. When it is not possible to achieve optimum conditions, this should be noted with the blood pressure reading, for example, "BP 154/92, R arm, V phase (patient very nervous)."

The defence reaction: "white coat hypertension"

Anxiety raises blood pressure, often by as much as 30 mm Hg. The defence or alarm reaction is a rise in blood pressure associated with blood pressure measurement. This increase may subside once the subject becomes accustomed to the procedure and the observer, but in many subjects blood pressure is always higher when measured by doctors, and to a lesser degree when measured by nurses—so called "white coat hypertension."

Points to bear in mind when measuring blood pressure

Explanation to subject

The first step, therefore, in blood pressure measurement is adequate explanation of the procedure in an attempt to allay fear and anxiety, especially in nervous subjects. In particular, subjects having blood pressure measured for the first time should be told that there is minor discomfort caused by inflation of the cuff.

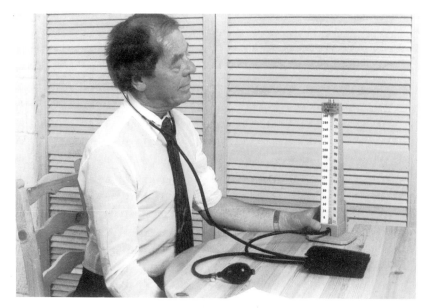

The observer should be aware of the physiological principles of blood pressure and be prepared to take the time necessary to achieve as accurate a measurement as possible. It takes about five minutes to measure the blood pressure accurately, although in practice considerably less time is devoted to the procedure.

Patient education

Many patients are anxious to learn more about high blood pressure and some are anxious to learn how to measure their own blood pressure; illustrated instruction books are helpful in this context.

Factors affecting blood pressure

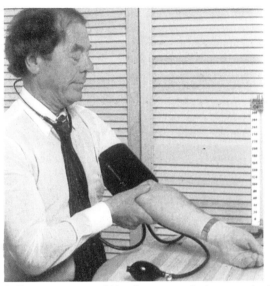
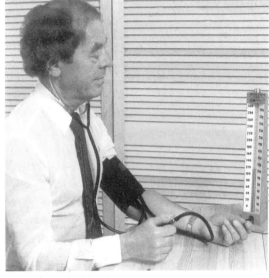

Self-measurement of blood pressure. Patients can be instructed to take blood pressure accurately using a mercury sphygmomanometer or an accurate automated device. (From O'Brien and O'Malley, 1987, with permission)

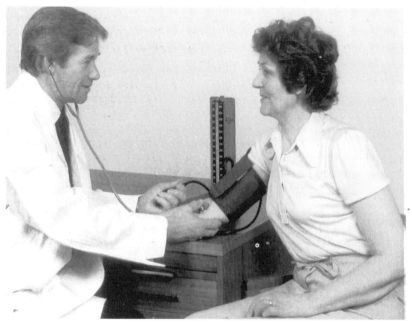

Seated subject with arm on table

Posture of subject

Posture affects blood pressure with a general tendency for it to increase from the lying to sitting or standing position. However, in most people posture is unlikely to lead to significant error in blood pressure measurement, provided the arm is supported at heart level. Nevertheless, it is advisable to standardise posture for individual patients and in practice blood pressure is usually measured in the sitting position. Patients should be comfortable whatever their position. No information is available on the optimal time that a subject should remain in a particular position before a measurement, but three minutes is suggested for the lying and sitting positions and one minute for standing. Some antihypertensive drugs cause postural hypotension and, when this is expected, blood pressure should be measured both lying and standing.

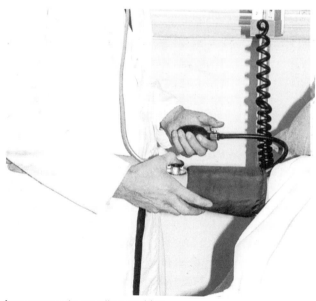
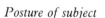

Arm support in standing position

Arm support

If the arm in which measurement is being made is unsupported, as tends to happen if the subject is sitting or standing, isometric exercise is performed thereby raising blood pressure and heart rate. Diastolic blood pressure may be raised by as much as 10% by having the arm extended and unsupported during blood pressure measurement. This effect of isometric exercise is greater in hypertensive patients and in those taking β blockers. It is therefore essential that the arm is supported during blood pressure measurement and this is best achieved in practice by having the observer hold the subject's arm at the elbow, although in research the use of an arm support on a stand has much to commend it.

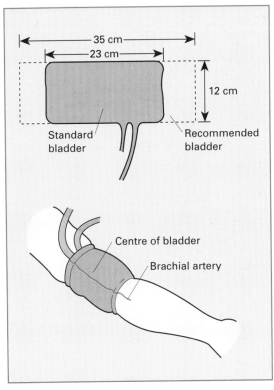

Correct placement of cuff and bladder

Arm position

The arm must also be horizontal at the level of the heart as denoted by the midsternal level. Positioning of the arm below heart level leads to an overestimation of systolic and diastolic pressures, and raising the arm above heart level leads to underestimation. The magnitude of this error can be as great as 10 mm Hg for both systolic and diastolic pressures. This source of error becomes particularly important in the sitting and standing positions when the arm is likely to be by the subject's side below heart level. It has been demonstrated, however, that even in the supine position an error of 5 mm Hg for diastolic pressure may occur if the arm is not supported at heart level.

Which arm

This topic remains controversial because some studies, although not all, using simultaneous measurement have demonstrated significant differences between arms (in as many as 5% of normotensive and 15% of hypertensive subjects).

A reasonable policy would be to measure blood pressure in both arms at the initial examination, and if differences of more than 20 mm Hg for systolic or 10 mm Hg for diastolic pressure are present on three consecutive readings simultaneous measurement should be carried out to determine whether the difference is real or artefactual. This is done by two trained observers recording the blood pressure simultaneously in both arms using one sphygmomanometer connected by a Y connector to the two occluding cuffs. In the absence of any cause for a difference, blood pressure should be recorded in the arm with the highest pressure.

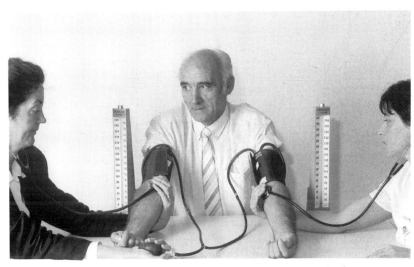

Technique for simultaneous measurement of blood pressure in both arms

The cuff should be wrapped round the arm ensuring that the bladder dimensions are accurate. If the bladder does not completely encircle the arm its centre must be over the brachial artery. The rubber tubes from the bladder are usually placed inferiorly, often at the site of the brachial artery, although it is now recommended that they should be placed superiorly or, with completely encircling bladders, posteriorly, so that the antecubital fossa is easily accessible for auscultation. The lower edge of the cuff should be 2–3 cm above the point of brachial artery pulsation.

Acknowledgement
O'Brien E, O'Malley K. *High blood pressure: what it means for you and how to control it.* London: Macdonald & Co., 1987:30–1.

Further reading
Mancia G, Parati G, Pomidossi G, Casadei R, Groppelli A, Sposato E, Zanchetti A. Doctor-elicited blood pressure rises at the time of sphygmomanometric blood pressure assessment persist over repeated visits. *J Hypertension* 1985;**3** (suppl 3):S421–3.
Pickering TG, James GD, Boddie C, Harshfield GA, Blank S, Laragh JH. How common is white coat hypertension? *JAMA* 1988;**2**:584–6.
O'Brien E, O'Malley K. Techniques for measuring blood pressure and their interpretation. In: Birkenhager W, ed. *Practical management of hypertension.* Dordrecht: Kluwer Academic Publishers, 1990.

BLOOD PRESSURE MEASUREMENT IN SPECIAL CIRCUMSTANCES

Obesity

Special circumstances
• Obesity
• Arrhythmias
• Children
• Pregnancy
• Elderly people

The association between obesity and hypertension has been recognised since 1923. The link has been confirmed in many epidemiological studies and has at least two components. First, there appears to be a pathophysiological connection and it may well be that in some cases the two conditions are causally linked; second, if not taken into account, it may result in inaccurate blood pressure values being obtained by indirect measurement techniques. The relationship of arm circumference and bladder dimension has been discussed in the previous chapter. In short, bladder length should be at least 80% of arm circumference. If the bladder is too short, blood pressure will be overestimated.

Many cuffs now bear marks that indicate the upper limit of arm circumference for which they are applicable. All physicians should have a large cuff (bladder dimensions 12×40 cm) available because obesity is quite commonly associated with raised blood pressure, and failure to take arm circumference into account may have serious implications for patient management. Generally, if bladder length is satisfactory, the error associated with width is small provided that the bladder width is at least 12 cm.

Arrhythmias

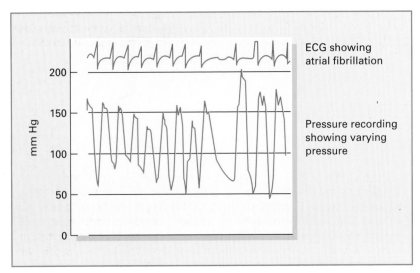

ECG showing atrial fibrillation

Pressure recording showing varying pressure

Arrhythmias and hypertension

The difficulty in measuring blood pressure in patients with arrhythmias is that when cardiac rhythm is irregular there is a large variation in blood pressure from beat to beat. Thus in arrhythmias, such as atrial fibrillation, stroke volume, and, as a consequence, blood pressures vary depending on the preceding pulse interval. Second, in such circumstances, there is no generally accepted method of determining auscultatory end points. The lack of a uniform approach is reflected by greater interobserver variability when blood pressure is measured in atrial fibrillation than when measured in sinus rhythm.

Some physicians may use the first Korotkov sound as systolic pressure whereas others may equate systolic pressure with the consistent presence of sounds. A similar problem pertains to interpreting diastolic blood pressure. If the first appearance of sound and the final disappearance of all sounds are taken to be systolic and diastolic blood pressure respectively, it seems likely that the systolic values will be overestimated and the diastolic values underestimated. Irrespective of what guidelines are agreed upon, blood pressure measurement in atrial fibrillation, particularly when the ventricular rhythm is highly irregular, will at best constitute a rough estimate, the validity of which can perhaps be improved upon only by using repeated measurements or direct intra-arterial measurement.

In bradyarrhythmias there may be two sources of error. First, if the rhythm is irregular the same problems as with atrial fibrillation will apply; second, when the heart rate is extremely slow, for example, 40 beats/min, it is important that the deflation rate used is less than for normal heart rates, because too rapid deflation will lead to underestimation of systolic and overestimation of diastolic pressure.

Children

Bladder sizes for children's cuffs

4 × 13 cm—small children

8 × 18 cm—young children

12 × 26 cm—older children

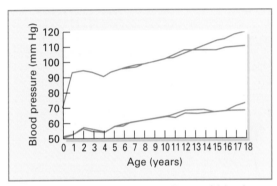

Mean systolic (top) and diastolic (bottom) blood pressures of boys and girls from birth to 18 years. Diastolic blood pressure reflects the use of phase IV Korotkov sounds. (From Whelton et al, 1989, with permission)

Blood pressure measurement in children presents a number of difficulties and variability of blood pressure is greater than in adults; thus any one reading is less likely to represent the true blood pressure. In addition, increased variability confers a greater tendency for regression towards the mean. Conventional sphygmomanometry is recomended for general use, although systolic pressure is preferred to diastolic because of the greater accuracy and reproducibility. Cuff dimensions are most important and three cuffs with bladders of the sizes in the box are required for the range of arm sizes likely to be encountered in the age range 0–14 years. The widest cuff practicable should be used. Korotkov sounds are not reliably audible in all children under one year and in many under five years of age. In such cases conventional sphygmomanometry is impossible and more sensitive methods of detection such as Doppler, ultrasonography, or oscillometry must be used.

Ideally blood pressure should be measured after a few minutes' rest. Values obtained during sucking, crying, or eating will not be representative. As with adults, a child's blood pressure status should only be decided after it has been measured on a number of separate occasions.

Between the ages of two and ten years normal blood pressure values are best related to height. In absolute terms blood pressure changes little within this age range. At age two years the mean blood pressure is 95 mm Hg with a 95th centile of 150 mm Hg. The corresponding values for the age of four days are 75 and 95 mm Hg respectively. Most children with blood pressure greater than the 95th centile are obese. After the age of 14 years adult norms should be used.

Pregnancy

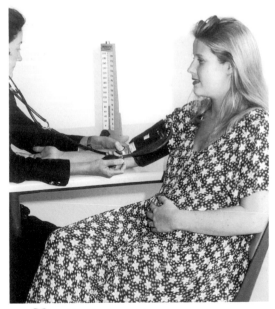

Measuring blood pressure in pregnancy

Between 2% and 5% of pregnancies in western Europe are complicated by clinically relevant hypertension and, in a significant number of these, raised blood pressure is a key factor in medical decision making in pregnancy. Particular attention must be paid to blood pressure measurement in pregnancy as a result of the important implications for patient management as well as the fact that it presents some special problems.

Various lines of approach have been used to predict the development of raised blood pressure in the last trimester, the most well known being the roll-over test. In this test an increase in the diastolic blood pressure of more than 20 mm Hg when the patient is turned from the lateral recumbent position to the supine position is considered a positive response. The test's value has been a matter of considerable controversy and it is not used much.

There has been much controversy over whether the muffling or disappearance of sounds should be taken for diastolic blood pressure. The general consensus now is that disappearance of sounds (fifth phase) is the most accurate measurement of diastolic pressure with the proviso that, if sounds persist to zero, the fourth phase of muffling of sounds should be used.

Twenty four hour ambulatory measurement is being used increasingly in pregnancy and is discussed on page 32.

13

Elderly people

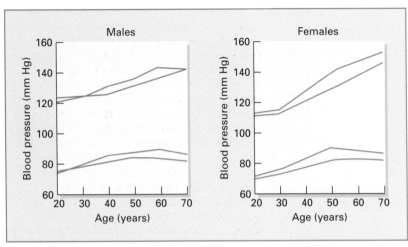

Age–blood pressure relationship by sex for systolic (top) and diastolic (bottom) blood pressures in the black (upper of two lines) and white (lower of two lines) general population of the United States of America, 1976–80. (Adapted from Whelton *et al*, 1989, with permission)

In epidemiological and interventional studies blood pressure predicts morbidity and mortality in elderly people as effectively as in the young. The extent to which it predicts outcome may be influenced by various factors that affect the accuracy of blood pressure measurement and the extent to which casual blood pressure represents the blood pressure load on the heart and circulation. Such difficulties may conveniently be considered in relation, first, to accuracy or validity of measurement and, second, to reliability of measurement which is affected by variability over time. Decreased accuracy or increased variability increases the likelihood of unrepresentative blood pressure values being used in clinical decision making and in research.

> **The standard technique for blood pressure measurement with a mercury sphygmomanometer is generally as accurate in elderly as in young patients.**

Accuracy

Of the pathophysiological changes that characterise hypertension in elderly people, none is more apparent than the tendency to have raised systolic blood pressure; this finds its extreme form in isolated systolic hypertension. There is a decrease in the elasticity and distensibility of the ageing blood vessels as a result of changes in smooth muscle proliferation and alterations in elastin, collagen, and calcium content. The structural and functional changes that occur with ageing are similar to those seen in hypertension itself. The combination of hypertension and ageing is manifest as a decrease in compliance. One consequence of this is the increase of systolic blood pressure found in elderly hypertensive individuals. A second consequence is that the decrease in compliance may interfere with the accuracy of indirect sphygmomanometry. This has led to the concept of "pseudohypertension" as a description of patients with a large discrepancy between cuff and direct blood pressure measurement.

Obesity is another factor that may adversely affect accuracy in elderly people. Although obesity may be present at any age, it is frequently a concomitant of hypertension in elderly people.

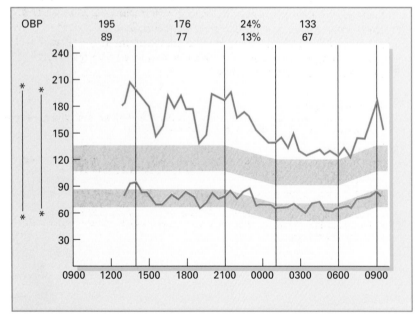

Isolated systolic hypertension in an elderly patient. Level of blood pressure is on the vertical axis and time of day on the horizontal axis. OBP is office blood pressure. In this patient the isolated elevation of blood pressure on OBP is sustained for the day period of a 24 hour recording and there is a 24/13% dip in nocturnal blood pressure.

Reliability

Blood pressure is subject to considerable variation from moment to moment as well as over days and years, making measurement relatively unreliable. As blood pressure variability increases in elderly people, measurement is even less reliable, and the likelihood of any one reading being representative of blood pressure diminishes. One way of reducing the impact of variability caused by factors such as diurnal patterns, white coat effect, anxiety, and cold is to carry out repeated measurements; this approach is particularly important in evaluating elderly patients. The value of repeated measurement is well illustrated by a reduction in the prevalence of isolated systolic hypertension from 13.9% to 2.7% on repeated blood pressure measurement. With the increasing use of ambulatory blood pressure measurement in assessment of hypertension in elderly people, it is beginning to emerge that many patients with apparent isolated systolic hypertension, when measured using conventional office blood pressure measurement, do not have sustained elevation of systolic blood pressure over the 24 hour period when using ambulatory techniques of measurement.

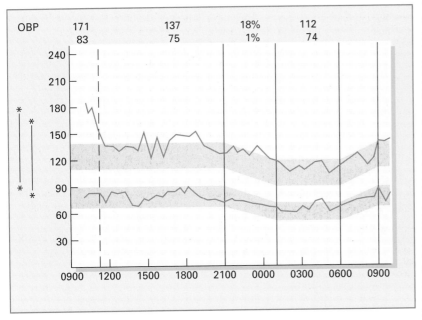

OBP	171	137	18%	112
	83	75	1%	74

In this patient, the isolated elevation of blood pressure on office blood pressure (OBP) is not sustained on the 24 hour recording

Postural and postprandial hypotension

Postural hypotension is more common in elderly people. It can coexist with raised supine and sitting blood pressure; it is therefore important that blood pressure be assessed in these positions as well as in the standing position on initial assessment, and from time to time in patients who are taking drugs known to cause postural hypotension.

Some elderly patients have quite a marked blood pressure fall after eating and this may be symptomatic. Again this can only be diagnosed definitively by measuring blood pressure when standing after a meal.

Autonomic failure is common in elderly people, and is best characterised by 24 hour blood pressure measurement which may show daytime hypotension when the subject is standing and night-time hypertension during recumbency.

> **Drugs known to cause postural hypotension include not only blood pressure lowering drugs, such as diuretics, but also non-cardiovascular drugs, for example, neuroleptics and tricyclic antidepressants.**

Acknowledgement
Whelton PK, Jiang H, Klag MJ. Blood pressure in Westernized populations. In: Swales, ed. *Textbook of hypertension*. Oxford: Blackwell Scientific Publications, 1994:14.

Further reading
de Swiet M, Dillon MJ, Littler W, O'Brien E, Padfield P, Petrie JC. Measurement of blood pressure in children. Recommendations of a Working Party of the British Hypertension Society. *BMJ* 1989;**299**:497.

O'Malley K, O'Brien E. Special clinical situations: the elderly. Messerli E, ed. *The ABCs of antihypertensive therapy*. New York: Raven Press, 1994;187–94.

O'Brien E, O'Malley K. Blood pressure measurement in the elderly with special reference to ambulatory blood pressure measurement. In: G Leonetti and Cuspedi, eds. *Hypertension in the elderly*. Dordrecht, Kluwer, 1994;13–25.

CONVENTIONAL BLOOD PRESSURE MEASUREMENT

THE OBSERVER

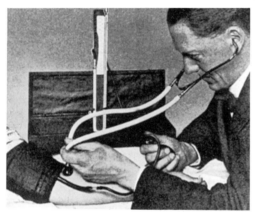

Riva-Rocci technique

The measurement of blood pressure in clinical practice by the century old technique of Riva-Rocci/Korotkov is dependent on the accurate transmission and interpretation of a signal (Korotkov sound or pulse wave) from a *subject* via a device (the *sphygmomanometer*) to an *observer*. The observer must be competent in performing the *technique* of blood pressure measurement, because it is the observer who has long been recognised as one of the major sources of error. There are two problems:

1. Deciding what constitutes adequate training
2. Devising a means of assessing the efficacy of training

Observer error

> **Rose's classification of observer error**
> - Systematic error
> - Terminal digit preference
> - Observer prejudice

In 1964, Geoffrey Rose and his colleagues classified observer error into three categories.

Systematic error

This leads to both intraobserver and interobserver error. It may be caused by lack of concentration, poor hearing, confusion of auditory and visual clues, etc. The most important factor is failure to interpret the Korotkov sounds accurately, especially for diastolic pressure.

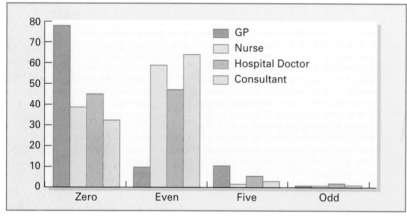

Diagram showing digit preference among different groups of observers for zero, even, odd, and five numerals in a large series from the Beaumont Hospital database

Terminal digit preference

This refers to the phenomenon whereby the observer rounds off the pressure reading to a digit of his or her choosing, most often to zero. GPs have a 12-fold bias in favour of the terminal digit zero; this has grave implications for decisions on diagnosis and treatment, although its greatest effect is in epidemiological and research studies in which it can distort the frequency distribution curve and reduce the power of statistical tests.

Observer prejudice or bias

This is the practice whereby the observer simply adjusts the pressure to meet his or her preconceived notion of what the pressure should be. It usually occurs when there has been recording of an excess of pressures below the cutoff point for hypertension and it reflects the observer's reluctance to diagnose hypertension. This is most likely to occur when an arbitrary division is applied between normal and high blood pressure, for example, 140/90 mm Hg. An observer might tend to record a favourable measurement in a young healthy man with a borderline increase in pressure, but categorise as hypertensive an obese, middle aged man with a similar reading. Likewise, there might be observer bias in overreading blood pressure to facilitate recruitment for a research project, such as a drug trial. Observer prejudice is a serious source of inaccuracy because the error cannot usually be demonstrated.

Training techniques

Observer training techniques

- Direct instruction by an experienced observer
- Instruction manuals and booklets
- Audio-tapes
- Video-films
- Computer instruction programs

It has been known from as far back as 1938, when the first survey of the "methods of teaching and interpretation" of blood pressure measurement was conducted, that discrepancies resulted in inadequate and inconsistent techniques of measurement. To achieve greater accuracy in observer performance, various methods and techniques have been used.

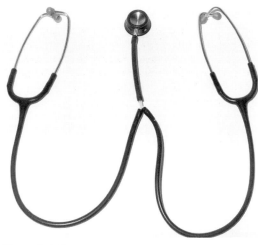

Binaural stethoscope

Direct instruction

Teaching the theory of blood pressure measurement has always been a feature of medical student and nursing education, but the practical demonstration of the technique traditionally takes place in the physiology class with the result that the student is not necessarily as competent measuring blood pressure as may be presumed. Nowadays, formal training probably constitutes part of the clinical curriculum in most medical and nursing schools; however, formal assessment of this skill is not always recognised as a prerequisite for the graduating physician or nurse.

The binaural stethoscope is an excellent instrument for both individual instruction and assessment of the accuracy of a trainee observer. Its disadvantage is that it only allows individual instruction, although modification of the technique has enabled use of a multiaural stethoscope to train as many as eight observers.

Examples of recommendations on measurement since 1986

- 1986: Petrie JC, O'Brien ET, Littler WA, de Swiet M. Recommendations on blood pressure measurement. British Hypertension Society. *BMJ* 1986; **293**: 611–15.
- 1988: Frohlich ED, Grim C, Labarthe DR, Maxwell MH, Perloff D, Weidman WH. Report of a Special Task Force Appointed by the Steering Committee, American Heart Association. Recommendations for the human blood pressure determination by sphygmomanometers. *Hypertension* 1988; **11**: 209A–22A.
- 1988: The Joint National Committee on the Detection, Evaluation, and Treatment of High Blood Pressure. The 1988 report of the Joint National Committee on the Detection, Evaluation, and Treatment of High Blood Pressure. *Arch Intern Med* 1988; **148**: 1023–38.
- 1988: Poggi L, Andre JL, Lyon A, Mallion JM, Plouin PF, Safar M. Mesure clinique de la pression arterielle: Recommendations. *Arch Mal Coeur* 1988; **81** (suppl HTA): 13–20.
- 1989: de Swiet M, Dillon MJ, Littler W, O'Brien E, Padfield P, Petrie JC. Measurement of blood pressure in children. Recommendations of a Working Party of the British Hypertension Society. *BMJ* 1989; **299**: 497.
- 1990: Specification for aneroid and mercury non-automated sphygmomanometers (Revision of BS 2743). British Standards Institution, London.
- 1990: Petrie JC, O'Brien ET, Littler WA, de Swiet M, Dillon MJ, Padfield PL. *Recommendations on blood pressure measurement.* BMJ Publishing Group, London, 2nd edn.
- 1991: Birkenhager WH, Reid JL, Series Eds, *Handbook of hypertension*, vol 14. O'Brien E, O'Mally K, Eds, *Blood pressure measurement.* Elsevier, Amsterdam.
- 1991: Pickering TG. *Ambulatory monitoring and blood pressure variability.* Science Press, London.
- 1994: *Ambulatory blood pressure.* Eds, H Brunner, B. Waeber. Raven Press, New York.

Manuals, booklets and published recommendations

The subject of blood pressure measurement has attracted interest since its introduction to clinical practice and this is reflected in a number of publications the purpose of which has been to improve observer technique and accuracy. These many publications clearly demonstrate the need for standardising blood pressure measurement techniques. In spite of this large number of recommendations, their effect in achieving better measurement has never been demonstrated. In fact, many nurses and doctors resent the implication that they might need to be trained or assessed in blood pressure measurement, with the result that most of the publications only influence a small number of those involved in such measurements. Those who read or peruse them are those who need them least – physicians with an interest in hypertension.

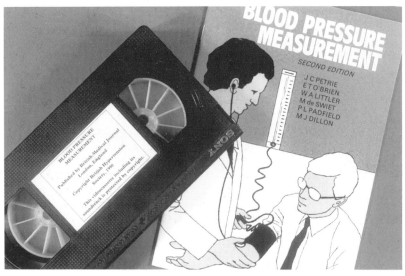

British Hypertension Society video and recommendations booklet

Audio-tape training methods

Audio-tape training methods make use of a set of stopwatches; these are stopped at systolic and diastolic end points, as determined by the Korotkov sounds for different pressures, played on a tape recording. This allows comparison between observers. If evidence of systematic error becomes evident in one or more observers, this can be demonstrated and hopefully eliminated by repeat sessions. Experience with audio-cassette tapes alone has, however, been disappointing.

Video-film methods

Videos and films consist of a series of blood pressure recordings in which a mercury column is seen falling in concert with recorded Korotkov sounds. The observer records the level of mercury in the column corresponding to the systolic and diastolic pressures. Within-observer reliability can be tested by duplication of recordings. The reference pressure is determined from the mean scores of a number of expert observers.

A video produced by the Working Party on Blood Pressure Measurement of the British Hypertension Society (BHS) incorporates this method; in addition, there is a visual presentation of the BHS recommendations on blood pressure measurement. Using this film and direct instruction it is possible to achieve nurse observer measurements among nurse observers that are within 5 mm Hg of each other.

Overcoming observer error

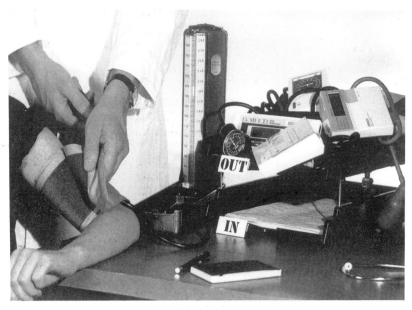

Validation of home devices. (From *Which?* August 1989, p. 372, with permission)

As mentioned earlier, blood pressure measurement is subject to observer prejudice and terminal digit preference, introducing an error that is unacceptable for research work, although careful training can greatly reduce this. The development of an accurate automated device would remove both observer prejudice and terminal digit preference; unfortunately, although there are many devices on the market, they have not been evaluated according to current requirements. Semiautomated devices for home measurement of blood pressure have failed to meet the required accuracy and performance criteria, but automated devices have recently achieved the standard of accuracy acceptable for clinical practice.

Two devices, based on the conventional technique, have been designed specifically for research use: the London School of Hygiene sphygmomanometer and the random zero sphygmomanometer. The first device, although popular in epidemiological studies for many years, had been accepted without validation as the "gold standard;" since 1982, when a calibration error was demonstrated, the device has not been in use.

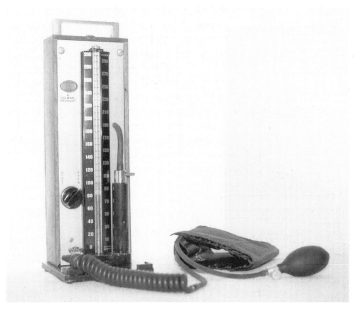
Hawksley random zero sphygmomanometer

The observer

In 1963, Garrow described a "zero-muddler for unprejudiced sphygmomanometry;" this was modified by Wright and Dore in 1970 and produced commercially by Hawksley and Sons. It had been generally accepted as the instrument of choice for epidemiological and research studies because it reduces observer bias and obscures digit preference, although the facility of the device to reduce terminal digit preference had been questioned. The accuracy of the random zero sphygmomanometer had been accepted rather uncritically, because it is basically a mercury sphygmomanometer, and it had replaced the London School of Hygiene Sphygmomanometer as the "gold standard." A number of recent studies have, however, demonstrated that the instrument systematically gives lower readings than the standard mercury sphygmomanometer, so it can no longer be recommended for accurate blood pressure measurement.

The development of more accurate semiautomated and automated devices should allow elimination of errors of interpretation together with observer bias and terminal digit preference. This apparent advance has, however, to be balanced against the considerable inaccuracy of many such devices. This is discussed further in the section on automated blood pressure measurement.

Observer training

Recommendations for observer training

Training observers in clinical practice

This includes nursing and medical students, doctors, and paramedical personnel

- Instruction in the theory of hypertension and blood pressure measurement
- Booklet for reading, for example, BHS *Recommendations on blood pressure measurement*
- Tutorial sessions with demonstrations using a binaural or multiaural stethoscope
- Video-film demonstration using, for example, the BHS video
- Video-film assessment
- Repeat video-film assessment until level of accuracy achieved
- Reassessment using BHS video-film every two years

Training observers in research

- Measurement of blood pressure — highest possible standard
- Level of accuracy
  90% of systolic and diastolic blood pressures within 5 mm Hg
  100% within 10 mm Hg of an expert observer
- Instruction in the theory of hypertension and blood pressure measurement
- Audiogram to check auditory acuity
- Booklet for reading, for example, BHS *Recommendations on blood pressure measurement*
- Tutorial sessions with demonstrations using a binaural or multiaural stethoscope
- Video-film demonstration using, for example, the BHS video
- Video-film assessment
- Repeat video-film assessment until level of accuracy achieved
- Training and assessment repeated at least every three months

To eliminate observer error a period of intensive training is needed, repeated at regular intervals if necessary, and it would be unrealistic to expect that such standards would be implemented in clinical practice. The criteria for observer accuracy are necessarily more stringent for research work than for clinical practice and recommendations for observer training have been drawn up for both.

Acknowledgement
Keep your blood pressure down. *Which?* August 1989, 372–5.

Further reading
Rose G. Standardisation of observers in blood-pressure measurement. *Lancet* 1965;i:673–4.
O'Brien E, Mee F, Tan KS, Atkins N, O'Malley K. Training and assessment of observers for blood pressure measurement. *J Hum Hypertens* 1991;5:7–10.
Curb JD, Labarthe DR, Poizner Cooper S, Cutter GR, Hawkins CM. Training and certification of blood pressure observers. *Hypertension* 1983;5:610–614.
Petrie J, Jamieson M, O'Brien E, Littler W, Padfield P, de Swiet M for the Working Party on Blood Pressure Measurement. Videotape *Blood pressure measurement*. London: BMJ Publishing Group, 1990.
Garrow JS. Zero-muddler for unprejudiced sphygmomanometry. *Lancet* 1963;iv:1205.
Rose GA, Holland WW, Crowley EA. A sphygmomanometer for epidemiologists. *Lancet* 1964;i:296–300.
Fitzgerald D, O'Callaghan W, O'Malley K, O'Brien E. Inaccuracy of the London School of Hygiene Sphygmomanometer. *BMJ* 1982;284:18–19.
O'Brien E, Mee F, Atkins N, O'Malley K. Inaccuracy of the Hawksley Random Zero Sphygmomanometer. *Lancet* 1990;336:1465–8.

MERCURY AND ANEROID SPHYGMOMANOMETERS

Two types of sphygmomanometer have been in common use since blood pressure measurement was first introduced: the mercury sphygmomanometer, which is a reliable device but all too often its continuing efficiency has been taken for granted, and the aneroid manometer, which is not generally as reliable. Both devices are used to measure blood pressure by auscultation using a stethoscope.

Standards are available from a number of national bodies, such as the British Standards Institution (BSI) and the Association for the Advancement of Medical Instrumentation (AAMI).

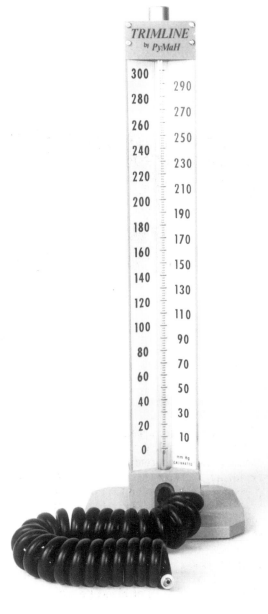

An example of a mercury sphygmomanometer

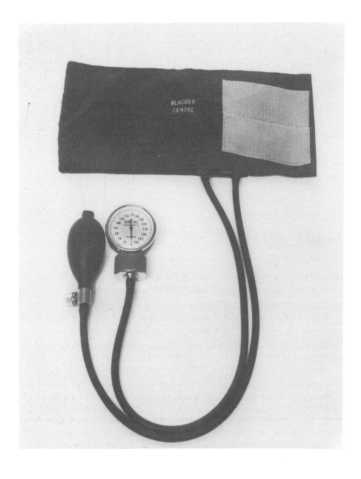

An example of an aneroid sphygmomanometer

Equipment

Consequences of defects in the control valve

Pumping control valve	Little or no effort required
Excessive squeeze on the pump	*Filter blocked*
With valve closed	Mercury at level steady
Falling mercury	*Leak in inflation system*
With valve released	Controlled fall of mercury
Failure to control mercury fall	*Leak in inflation system*

Control valve

One of the most common sources of error in sphygmomanometers is the control valve, especially when an air filter rather than a rubber valve is used. Defective valves cause leakage, making control of pressure release difficult; this leads to underestimation of systolic and overestimation of diastolic pressures. Faults in the control valve may be corrected easily and cheaply, by simply cleaning the filter or replacing the control valve. It is helpful to have a checklist of possible faults and the means of rectifying these.

How to test the control valve

- Roll a cloth cuff into its own tail
  Roll a Velcro cuff, matching Velcro to Velcro
- Pump up to 200 mm Hg and wait for 10 seconds
- Mercury should fall < 2 mm Hg in 10 seconds
- If fall > 2 mm Hg clamp circuit in sections to locate leak
- Failure: usually control valve
- Replace control valve
- Release valve slowly four times
  On two of four releases rate should be controlled to fall 1 mm Hg/s
  Easy to change from fast to slow rates
- Failure: usually blockage of air filter in the valve
- Clean filter

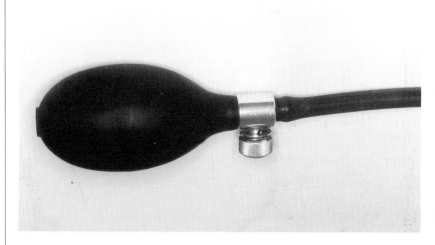

Hand pump and control valve

Features affecting accuracy of the mercury sphygmomanometer

- The top of the mercury meniscus should rest at exactly zero with no pressure applied; if it is below this add mercury
- The scale should be clearly calibrated in 2 mm divisions from 0 to 300 mm Hg and should indicate accurately the differences between the levels of mercury in the tube and in the reservoir
- The diameter of the reservoir must be at least 10 times that of the vertical tube, or the vertical scale must correct for the drop in the mercury level in the reservoir as the column rises
- Substantial errors may occur if the manometer is not kept vertical during measurement. Calibrations on floor models are specially adjusted to compensate for the tilt in the face of the gauge. Stand mounted manometers are recommended for hospital use. This allows the observer to adjust the level of the sphygmomanometer and to perform measurement without having to balance the sphygmomanometer precariously on the side of the bed
- The air vent at the top of the manometer must be kept patent because clogging will cause the mercury column to respond sluggishly to pressure changes and to overestimate pressure
- The control valve is one of the most common sources of error in sphygmomanometers and when it becomes defective it should be replaced. Spare control valves should be available in hospitals and a spare control valve should be supplied with sphygmomanometers

Mercury sphygmomanometers

The mercury sphygmomanometer is the simplest, most accurate, and most economical device for the indirect measurement of blood pressure; it is the device that is currently recommended for the clinical measurement of blood pressure. It can be maintained and serviced easily without having to be returned to the supplier but users should be alert to the hazards associated with handling mercury. A review of the features that are relevant to the clinical measurement of blood pressure is given in the box.

Mercury and aneroid sphygmomanometers

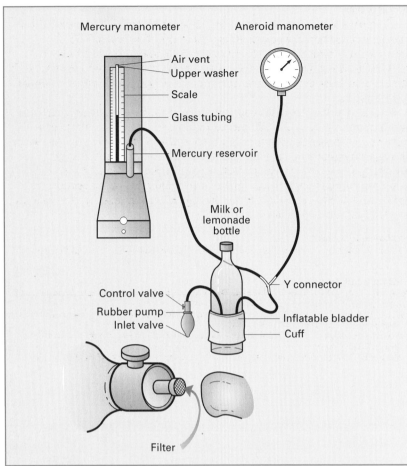

Method for calibrating an aneroid sphygmomanometer (from O'Brien and O'Malley, 1981)

Aneroid manometers

Aneroid sphygmomanometers register pressure through a bellows and lever system which is mechanically more intricate than the mercury reservoir and column. Their accuracy is affected by the jolts and bumps of everyday use; they lose accuracy over time usually leading to falsely low readings with the consequent underestimation of blood pressure. They are less accurate than mercury sphygmomanometers. When calibrated against a mercury sphygmomanometer a mean difference of 3 mm Hg is considered to be acceptable; however, 30–35% of aneroid sphygmomanometers have an average difference of more than 3 mm Hg, and some 6–13% deviate by 7 mm Hg or more.

Aneroid sphygmomanometers must be checked every six months against an accurate mercury sphygmomanometer over the entire pressure range, which can be done by connecting the aneroid sphygmomanometer via a Y piece to the tubing of the mercury sphygmomanometer and inflating the cuff around a bottle or cylinder. If inaccuracies or other faults are found, the instrument must be returned to the manufacturer or supplier for repair.

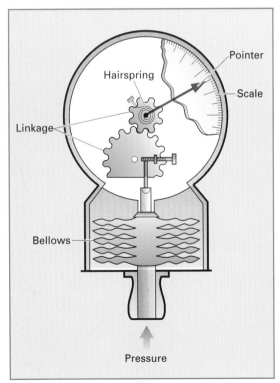

Mechanism of an aneroid sphygmomanometer

Stethoscope

A stethoscope should be of a high quality, in good condition, and with clean, well fitting ear pieces. The American Heart Association recommends using the bell of the stethoscope over the brachial artery rather than placing the diaphragm over the antecubital fossa, based on the fact that the bell is most suited to the auscultation of low pitched sounds, such as the Korotkov sounds. However, it probably does not matter much whether the bell or diaphragm is used in routine blood pressure measurement, provided that the stethoscope is placed over the palpated brachial artery in the antecubital fossa. As the diaphragm covers a greater area and is easier to hold than a bell end piece, it is reasonable to recommend it for routine clinical measurement of blood pressure, but in research work, where every effort should be made to achieve maximal accuracy, the bell rather than the diaphragm is preferred.

Helpful points for maintenance

- Booklet from manufacturers with recommendations for maintenance
- Warning of risks of mercury spillage
- Instructions for dealing with mercury spillage
- Agency/engineer responsible for maintenance
- Date of last maintenance/calibration
- Date when next maintenance/calibration due

Maintenance

Mercury sphygmomanometers are easily checked and maintained but care should be taken when handling mercury. The revised BHS Standard recommends that mercury sphygmomanometers display a warning to this effect. Mercury sphygmomanometers need cleaning and checking at least every six months in hospital use and every 12 months in general use.

As many as half the sphygmomanometers in hospital use are defective and a maintenance policy should be mandatory in all hospitals. Few have any such policy. Doctors in practice also often neglect having their sphygmomanometers checked and serviced. The responsibility for reporting faulty equipment or lack of appropriate cuffs lies with the observer, who should always refuse to use defective or inappropriate equipment. The responsibility for arranging regular maintenance should be clearly defined for each clinical area.

Acknowledgement

[1] O'Brien E, O'Malley K. *Essentials of blood pressure measurement.* Edinburgh: Churchill Livingstone, 1981.

Further reading

Burke MJ, Towers H, O'Malley K, Fitzgerald DJ, O'Brien ET. Sphygmomanometers in hospital and family practice: problems and recommendations. *BMJ* 1982;285:469–71.
Conceico S, Ward MK, Kerr DNS. Defects in sphygmomanometers: an important source of error in blood pressure recording. *BMJ* 1979;i:886–8.
Perlman LV, Chiang BN, Keller J, Blackburn H. The accuracy of sphygmomenometers. *Arch Intern Med* 1970;125:1000–3.
Bowman CE. Blood pressure errors with aneroid sphygmomanometers. *Lancet* 1981;i:1005.

TECHNIQUE OF AUSCULTATORY BLOOD PRESSURE MEASUREMENT

Techniques

> - The manometer should be no further than 3 feet or 1 metre away so that the scale can be read easily
> - The mercury column should be vertical (some models are designed with a tilt) and at eye level — this is achieved most effectively with stand mounted models which can be easily adjusted to suit the height of the observer
> - The mercury manometer has a vertical scale and errors will occur unless the eye is kept close to the level of the meniscus. The aneroid scale is a composite of vertical and horizontal divisions and numbers, and must be viewed straight on with the eye on a line perpendicular to the centre of the face of the gauge

Attitude of observer
Before taking the blood pressure, the observer should be in a comfortable and relaxed position, because if hurried the pressure will be relased too rapidly, resulting in underestimation of systolic and overestimation of diastolic pressures. If any interruption occurs the exact measurement may be forgotten and an approximation made, so always write down the blood pressure as soon as it has been measured.

Position of manometer
The observer should take care about positioning the manometer (see box).

Palpatory estimation of blood pressure
The brachial artery should be palpated while the cuff is rapidly inflated to about 30 mm Hg above the point where the pulse disappears; the cuff is then slowly deflated, and the observer notes the pressure at which the pulse reappears. This is the approximate level of the systolic pressure. Palpatory estimation is important because phase I sounds sometimes disappear as pressure is reduced and reappear at a lower level (the auscultatory gap), resulting in systolic pressure being underestimated unless already determined by palpation. The palpatory technique is useful in patients in whom auscultatory end points may be difficult to judge accurately — for example, pregnant women, patients in shock, or those taking exercise. (The radial artery is often used for palpatory estimation of the systolic pressure but by using the brachial artery the observer also establishes its location before auscultation.)

Manometer level in relation to the eye of the observer

Auscultatory measurement of systolic and diastolic pressures
- Place the stethoscope gently over the brachial artery at the point of maximal pulsation; a bell end piece gives better sound reproduction although, for clinical practice, a diaphragm is easier to secure with the fingers of one hand and covers a larger area.
- The stethoscope should be held firmly and evenly but without excessive pressure — too much pressure may distort the artery, producing sounds below diastolic pressure. The stethoscope end piece should not touch the clothing, cuff, or rubber tubes to avoid friction sounds.

- The cuff should then be inflated rapidly to about 30 mm Hg above the palpated systolic pressure and deflated at a rate of 2–3 mm Hg/pulse beat (or per second) during which the auscultatory phenomena will be heard.
- When all sounds have disappeared the cuff should be deflated rapidly and completely before repeating the measurement to prevent venous congestion of the arm. The phases shown in the box, which were first described by Nicolai Korotkov and later elaborated by Witold Ettinger, are heard during the procedure.

Auscultatory sounds

- *Phase I*: the first appearance of faint, repetitive, clear tapping sounds which gradually increase in intensity for at least two consecutive beats is the systolic blood pressure
- *Phase II*: a brief period may follow during which the sounds soften and acquire a swishing quality
- *Auscultatory gap*: in some patients sounds may disappear altogether for a short time
- *Phase III*: the return of sharper sounds, which become crisper to regain, or even exceed, the intensity of phase I sounds. The clinical significance, if any, of phases II and III has not been established
- *Phase IV*: the distinct abrupt muffling of sounds, which become soft and blowing in quality
- *Phase V*: the point at which all sounds finally disappear completely is the diastolic pressure

---

Diastolic dilemma

For many years recommendations on blood pressure measurement have been uncertain about the diastolic end point — the so called "diastolic dilemma." Phase IV (muffling) may coincide with or be as much as 10 mm Hg higher than phase V (disappearance), but usually the difference is less than 5 mm Hg; phase V correlates best with intra-arterial pressure. There has been resistance to general acceptance of the silent end point until recently, because the silent end point can be greatly below the muffling of sounds in some groups of patients — children, pregnant women, anaemic, or elderly patients. In some patients sounds may even be audible when cuff pressure is deflated to zero. There is now a general consensus that disappearance of sounds (phase V) should be taken as diastolic pressure except in those subjects mentioned above (as originally recommended by Korotkov in 1910). In 1962 the World Health Organization recommended, with support from others, that both phases IV and V should be recorded.

Recording blood pressure

The points to be noted when measuring blood pressure are listed in the box.

Number of measurements

One measurement should be taken carefully at each visit, with a repeat measurement if there is uncertainty or distraction; do not make a number of hurried measurements.

As a result of the variability of measurements of casual blood pressure, decisions based on single measurements will result in erroneous diagnosis and inappropriate management. Reliability of measurements is improved if repeat measurements are made. The alarm reaction to blood pressure measurement may persist after several visits, so for patients in whom sustained increases of blood pressures are being assessed, a number of measurements should be made on different occasions over a number of weeks or months before diagnostic or management decisions are made.

What to note when measuring blood pressure

- The blood pressure should be written down as soon as it has been recorded
- Measurement of systolic and diastolic pressure should be made to the nearest 2 mm Hg
- Pressures should not be rounded off to the nearest 5 or 10 mm Hg — digit preference
- The arm in which the pressure is being recorded and the position of the subject should be noted
- Pressures should be recorded in both arms on first attendance
- In obese patients the bladder size should be indicated
- If a "standard" cuff containing a bladder with the dimensions 23×12 cm has to be used in subjects with large arm circumferences, it is best to state this together with the measurement, so that the presence of "cuff hypertension" can be taken into account in diagnostic and management decisions, and arrangements can be made for a more accurate measurement
- In clinical practice the diastolic pressure should be recorded as phase V, except in those patients in whom sounds persist greatly below muffling; this should be clearly indicated
- In hypertension research both phases IV and V should be recorded
- If the patient is anxious, restless, or distressed, and this influences blood pressure behaviour, a note should be made with the blood pressure
- The presence of an auscultatory gap should always be indicated
- In patients taking drugs that lower blood pressure the optimal time for control of blood pressure will depend on the timing of the drug administration; when assessing the effect of antihypertensive drugs the time of drug ingestion should be noted in relation to the time of measurement
- The following are examples of comprehensive recordings of blood pressure in two clinical situations:
  — R. arm 154/82; L. 148/76; phase V; 26 cm bladder; sitting; subject anxious; no medication
  —R. arm 210/52; L. arm 204/48; phase IV/auscultatory gap; 40 cm bladder; AC 38 cm; lying; medication at 08:00 hours/BP at 09:30 hours

---

Further reading
Short D. The diastolic dilemma. *BMJ* 1975;ii:685–6.
London SB, London RE. Critique of indirect diastolic end point. *Arch Intern Med* 1967;**119**:39–49.
Folsom AR, Prineas RJ, Jacobs DR, Luepker RV, Gillum RF. Measured differences between fourth and fifth phase diastolic blood pressures in 4885 adults: implications for blood pressure surveys. *Int J Epidemiol* 1984;**13**:436–41.
King GE. Recommendations for sphygmomanometry. A dissenting opinion. *Am Heart J* 1969;**77**:147–8.
Manek S, Rutherford J, Jackson SHD, Turner P. Persistence of divergent views of hospital staff in detecting and managing hypertension. *BMJ* 1984;**289**:1433–4.
Hense H-W, Stieber J, Chambless L. Factors associated with measured differences between fourth and fifth phase diastolic blood pressure. *Int J Epidemiol* 1986;**15**:513–18.

AUTOMATED BLOOD PRESSURE MEASUREMENT

SEMIAUTOMATED AND AUTOMATED DEVICES

One consequence of the increased interest in blood pressure measurement has been the creation of a large market for blood pressure measuring devices. In recent years the number of devices available commercially has risen rapidly but many have been shown to be inaccurate when compared with the mercury sphygmomanometer; recently there have been promising signs that we may soon have a selection of accurate and inexpensive automated devices.

Principles of automated measurement

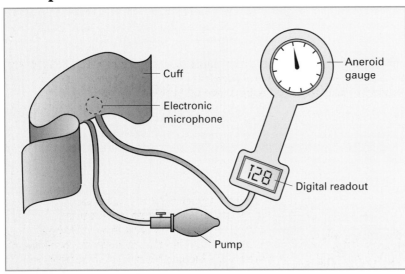

Diagram of a simple semiautomated sphygmomanometer; most recent devices incorporate automated inflation/deflation, a digital display, and print out

Most semiautomated devices work on one of three principles: the detection of Korotkov sounds by a microphone or the detection of arterial blood flow by either ultrasonography or oscillometry. Until recently semiautomated devices depended on the detection of Korotkov sounds using an electronic microphone shielded from extraneous noise in the pressure cuff, with blood pressure being recorded on a print out or indicated on a digital display. The microphones are sensitive to movement and friction, however, and may be difficult to place accurately. Manufacturers are turning, therefore, to oscillometric detection of blood pressure in which cuff placement is not critical. Manual or automatic inflation and deflation, or both, may be available. Other techniques have been tried or are being developed, but as with other automated devices the results of validation have often been disappointing.

Complex devices that record blood pressure automatically at preset intervals have been designed for intensive care units and operating rooms and these often use two methods of measurement, most commonly detection of Korotkov sounds and oscillometry. Often, however, the mode is not indicated, assessments of accuracy are not always available from the manufacturers, and some devices are difficult to assess independently. Comparison of results is difficult and it may be many years before there is sufficient evidence on which to make a confident judgment.

Techniques for measuring blood pressure

- Microphonic detection of Korotkov's sounds
- Oscillometry
- Ultrasonography
- Phase shift method
- Infrasound recording
- Wide band external pulse recording
- Plethysmography
- Tonometry

Validation of 10 self measuring devices

Devices not fulfilling the BHS protocol for accuracy

Omron HEM-400C	Philips HP5308
Philips HP5306	Phillips HP5332
Healthcheck CX-5	Systema DrMI-150
Nissei BPM	Nissei DS-175
Fortec DrMI-100	

Device fulfilling the BHS protocol for accuracy
Omron HEM-705CP

Self measuring semiautomated devices validated by one laboratory over a five year period; only the Omron HEM-705CP fulfilled the accuracy criteria of the British Hypertension Society protocol.

Similarities with conventional measurement

Principles of measurement common to conventional measurement

- The cuff and bladder
- Inflation–deflation system
- Standards for blood pressure measuring devices
- Factors common to the subject
- Blood pressure measurement in special circumstances

The use of automated devices is governed by many of the principles that apply to conventional measurement using the mercury sphygmomanometer.

Self (home) measurement

Since Brown's observation in 1930 that blood pressure measured in the home was lower than that recorded by a doctor, the discrepancy between pressures recorded in the home and the clinic has been confirmed repeatedly, and this is the case whether measured by patients, or their relatives or friends.

- Training the patient to measure blood pressure is troublesome, although a satisfactory degree of competence can probably be achieved by using illustrated instructions
- Subjective bias whereby the patient notes pressures that he or she might desire to record
- The technique may cause anxiety or cause the patient to take an obsessional interest in blood pressure
- Most devices available for self measurement have not been validated adequately or have been shown to be inaccurate

Why then has home measurement of blood pressure failed to achieve the success and popularity of home urinalysis in diabetes? There are a number of explanations (as listed in the box).

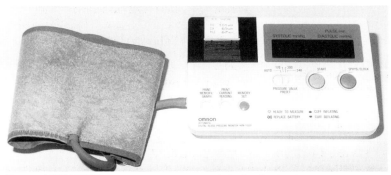

The Omron HEM-705CP: an accurate automated device for blood pressure measurement which provides a print out with the time and date of measurement

For the reasons in the box, home measurement of blood pressure has not received widespread acceptance, although it is useful in carefully selected patients. A 24 hour ambulatory blood pressure measurement (see the next chapter) is becoming the preferred method of assessing blood pressure behaviour because this provides a more objective blood pressure profile which is also free of bias. The advent of accurate inexpensive automated devices which can provide a printout of blood pressure measurement with time and date would remove many of the drawbacks referred to above and may lead to increased use of this technique.

Further reading

O'Brien E, Atkins N, Mee F, O'Malley K. Inaccuracy of seven popular sphygmomanometers for home-measurememt of blood pressure. *J Hypertens* 1990;8:621–34.

Pickering TG, Cvetkovski B, James GD. An evaluation of electronic recorders for self-motivating of blood pressure. *J Hypertens* 1986;4(suppl 5):S328–30.

Evans CE, Haynes RB, Goldsmith CH, Hewson SA. Home blood pressure-measuring devices: a comparative study of accuracy. *J Hypertens* 1989;7:133–42.

Steiner R, Luscher T, Boerlin H-J, Siegenthaler W, Vetter W. Clinical evaluation of semiautomatic blood pressure devices for self-recording. *J Hypertens* 1985;3(suppl):23–5.

AMBULATORY BLOOD PRESSURE MEASUREMENT

- Accuracy of the devices
- Normal reference values of 24 hour pressure
- Relationship of ABPM to cardiovascular morbidity

The first intra-arterial ambulatory blood pressure measurement (ABPM) was performed in Oxford in 1966; using this system it soon became apparent that blood pressure varied considerably in response to a variety of stresses, including the presence of a doctor, nurse, or technician, lecturing, driving a motor car, and having sexual intercourse. Furthermore, ABPM made it possible to determine, not only the blood pressure lowering efficacy of antihypertensive drugs, but also their duration of action. Most excitingly of all, perhaps, 24 hour ambulatory recordings provided enough data for the characterisation of nocturnal blood pressure and the diurnal pattern of blood pressure.

Much research and technological development over the past 25 years has resulted in the manufacture of ambulatory systems which do not depend on intra-arterial measurement. As they are non-invasive and almost completely free of adverse effects, these systems have found much wider use in research and clinical practice than was ever possible with invasive techniques. ABPM will probably become indispensable in the assessment of patients with elevated blood pressure. Three fundamental issues need to be examined, however, before the technique can be permitted to pass from research to clinical practice, as listed in the box.

Accuracy of ambulatory systems?

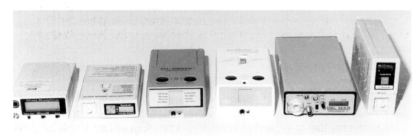

A selection of the many ambulatory systems now on the market

There are at least 30 ABPM systems now available with many more in the development phase. To ensure that ambulatory systems are accurate and perform satisfactorily in clinical practice, the BHS Working Party on Blood Pressure Measurement published a comprehensive protocol for the evaluation of blood pressure measuring devices. This incorporates some of the validation criteria of the Association for the Advancement of Medical Instrumentation (AAMI), together with many additional aspects.

Data for nine ABPM systems which have been evaluated using the BHS and AAMI protocols are shown in the box.

ABPM devices that have fulfilled BHS* and AAMI** accuracy criteria

Manufacturer	Device	Mechanism
Disetronic Medical Systems	CH-Druck	Auscultatory
	Profilomat	Auscultatory
IDT	Nissei DS-240	Auscultatory Oscillometric
Welch Allyn	Quiet Track	Auscultatory
SpaceLabs Inc	SpaceLabs 90202	Oscillometric
	SpaceLabs 90207	Oscillometric
A&D Company	TM-2420 Model 6	Auscultatory
	TM-2420 Model 7	Auscultatory
	TM-2421	Oscillometric

Assessment took place in January 1995
* Criteria: devices must achieve at least grade B/B.
** Criteria: mean difference <5 mmHg (SD<8 mmHg).

BHS grading criteria

	Grade	mm Hg absolute difference between standard and test device		
		≤5	≤10	≤15
Cumulative	A	60	85	95
(% of	B	50	75	90
readings)	C	40	65	85
	D	Worse than C		

Grades are derived from percentages of readings within 5, 10 and 15 mm Hg. To achieve a grade all three percentages must be equal to or greater than the tabulated values.

Each evaluation was performed under standardised conditions to allow comparison of devices, and the results are shown in the table which allows comparison of accuracy.

Normal values for ABPM

To establish ABPM in clinical practice, it is necessary to establish normal reference values for blood pressure levels. There are two basic approaches to defining normalcy for 24 hour ABPM.

Relationship of ABPM to morbidity, mortality, and target organ involvement

The classic epidemiological approach is the establishment of a relationship to the risk of heart attack, stroke, and death in longitudinal studies. There has, however, only been one such study performed to date — as first reported by Sokolow's group in 1964; this shows that ABPM predicts cardiovascular risk better than clinical blood pressure.

If the relationship of ABPM to end organ involvement is substituted for the classic end points of death and morbidity, it is possible for an association with risk to be demonstrated in a shorter period of time.

In all such studies ABPM correlates better with target organ damage than conventional blood pressure measurement.

Upper limits of normal for ABPM in normotensive subjects in three large population studies

	Number	Conventional pressure	Ambulatory pressure		
			24 h	Day	Night
Belgian population	574	139/90	132/82	140/89	123/74
Irish (AIB) population	806	139/91	132/83	142/91	123/74
International database	4577	143/91	136/84	144/91	128/77

ABPM levels in normal populations

An alternative option is to determine the distribution of 24 hour blood pressures in normal population or community samples which define levels according to centiles or standard deviations above or below the mean values for a given population. Reference tables showing normal levels for different ages and sex have been produced; using the data from the Allied Irish Bank (AIB) study it is possible to produce a working definition of normalcy. Allowances should be made for the considerable differences for age and gender shown by the AIB study.

A number of population studies have now been conducted in different countries and there is reassuring consistency among these studies as to what constitutes normality. The Belgian and the Irish AIB population studies yield almost identical upper limits of normalcy for ABPM. A large international database analysis incorporating 4577 subjects from different countries yielded slightly higher systolic pressures, reflecting the slightly higher pressures at entry when blood pressure was measured using the conventional technique. These large samples allow for the establishment of operational thresholds for ABPM in clinical practice as shown in the box.

Mean (±SD) office and 24 hour ambulatory blood pressure in 815 people according to age and sex in the Allied Irish Bank Study

		Men				All	Women				All	Both
Age range		17–29	30–39	40–49	50–79	17–79	17–29	30–39	40–49	50–79	17–79	17–79
n		107	123	109	60	399	174	149	55	38	416	815
Office measurements												
	SBP	121±12	122±11	125±16	133±15	124±14	110±11	113±10	121±17	130±24	115±15	119±15
	DBP	73±9	77±8	81±10	85±11	78±10	71±8	72±8	78±9	81±12	73±9	76±10
Ambulatory measurements												
Day	SBP	129±8	128±9	129±12	132±12	129±10	118±8	117±8	121±12	126±18	118±10	124±12
	DBP	77±7	80±6	83±9	84±9	81±8	74±6	75±7	76±9	78±9	75±7	78±8
Night	SBP	110±9	108±8	109±12	113±13	110±10	102±9	101±9	103±11	108±12	102±9	106±11
	DBP	59±6	62±6	66±10	68±9	63±8	57±6	58±7	61±8	63±7	58±7	61±8
24 hour	SBP	123±8	121±8	122±11	126±12	123±10	112±7	111±8	114±10	120±15	113±9	118±11
	DBP	71±5	74±5	77±8	79±9	75±7	68±5	69±6	71±8	73±8	69±6	72±7

SBP, DBP, systolic and diastolic pressures (mm Hg), respectively.

Indications for ABPM in clinical practice

As we enter the last decade of this century one fact is clear—ABPM is passing from research to clinical practice and it behoves us to ensure that it is not misused in this capacity by providing adequate guidelines.

The introduction of ABPM to clinical practice is proceeding at a rapid pace. In at least six European countries ambulatory devices are becoming available in general practice. The impetus for introducing a new development to clinical practice often derives from market rather than from scientific considerations, and the pharmaceutical companies are at the forefront in the propagation of ABPM in general practice.

ABPM operator requirements

- Familiarity with the equipment
- Knowledge of the calibration procedures for the device
- Knowledge about the normal ranges of blood pressure during the day and night
- Awareness of the factors influencing the diurnal pattern
- Giving the necessary time to instruct the subject so as to obtain as many measurements as possible during the recording period
- Subjects for ABPM must be capable of coping with and caring for the recorder
- Conditions of measurement for the subject should be standardised as far as possible:
    Subject's arm should be still during measurement
    Similar levels of activity for comparative repeat measurements
    Working days should not be compared with recreational days
    Comparative measurements in shift workers should be made between similar shifts
- For clinical use recordings are usually programmed for every 30 minutes
- Subjects should keep a diary of activities and symptoms during the recording period

Device and operator requirements

Ambulatory systems must be accurate and reasonably priced, with recorders that are compact, noiseless, light, and comfortable for the patient to wear. In obese subjects a cuff containing an appropriately sized bladder must be used.

The operator must be familiar with certain basic principles.

The clinical indications for using ABPM are best considered in relation to the diagnosis of hypertension, and the selection and evaluation of antihypertensive drug treatment.

Diagnosis

Using ABPM in clinical practice enables a more accurate diagnosis to be made. In particular normalcy over 24 hours can be determined, "white coat hypertension" can be excluded, and non-dippers can be identified.

Normalcy—The normal ranges for ABPM for adults have been defined according to sex and age; it is now possible to plot 24 hour pressures for each patient and determine whether they fall within the normal bands using either two standard deviations or 5th and 95th centiles to define the upper and lower limits of pressure.

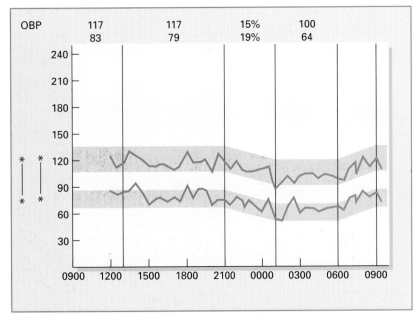

Plot of normal ABPM: office blood pressure (OBP=conventional blood pressure) is shown before the vertical axis for blood pressure level; time of day is on the horizontal axis; the shaded bands indicate the upper and lower limits of 24 hour blood pressure as determined in the AIB Study. The first vertical line closes the "white coat" window when the effect of medical staff on blood pressure may be still evident; the second line closes the daytime period; the third line closes the retiring window when pressures fall before settling for the night time period, which is closed by the fourth veritcal line, and the last vertical line closes the awakening window when pressures start to rise. The levels of blood pressure for the successive windows and the nocturnal dip in blood pressure are shown above. All records have been taken from the Beaumont Hospital Blood Pressure database and are unedited

Diagnostic indications for ABPM

- "White coat hypertension"
- Borderline hypertension
- Isolated systolic hypertension in elderly people
- Nocturnal dipper status
- Evaluation of hypotensive symptoms
- Miscellaneous diagnostic uses

The following patients benefit most from ABPM and should be referred for the procedure, at least on initial assessment. The identification of subjects with white coat hypertension is the most important clinical indication for ambulatory measurement.

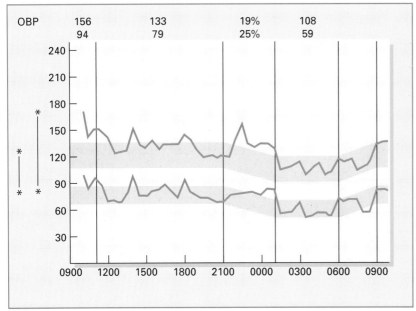

Plot of white coat hypertension. The elevation of OBP is carried into the "white coat window" but thereafter pressures are within the normal bands with 19/25% nocturnal dip in pressure

"White coat hypertension"—This may be defined simply as a rise in blood pressure associated with the procedure of having blood pressure measured. It may result partly from anxiety, although in many subjects there is a deeper "learning" process whereby the centres subserving blood pressure control have been conditioned to elevate blood pressure for the procedure of measurement. Whatever the mechanism, the reality is that as many as 20% of patients labelled as having "hypertension" using conventional blood pressure measurement may have "white coat hypertension" and may not therefore require blood pressure lowering drugs. ABPM is the most effective method of determining whether blood pressure elevation is the result of the white coat effect.

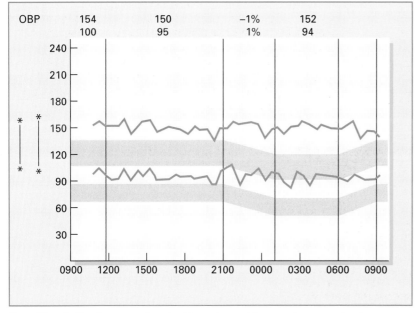

Plot of borderline hypertension. In this patient white coat hypertension is excluded as the cause for elevation of OBP, and all the 24 hour pressures are clearly elevated with a non-dipping nocturnal profile

Borderline hypertension—ABPM is particularly helpful in deciding whether subjects with borderline elevation of clinic/office blood pressure, who may be subjected to unnecessary treatment or penalised for insurance cover and employment, should be labelled as hypertensive. In practice, this means that all newly diagnosed hypertensive patients should have their 24 hour profile characterised; this should certainly be done before antihypertensive drugs are prescribed. In subjects with borderline hypertension and evidence of target organ involvement, but in whom ABPM is normal, hypertension may be excluded as a cause for the target organ damage.

"White coat hypertension" may not be innocent

- Patients whose blood pressures are elevated in the presence of a doctor or in the medical environment, although not necessarily needing antihypertensive treatment, should not be dismissed as "normal"
- There is some evidence that the "white coat phenomenon" is an early manifestation of haemodynamic disturbance and that patients may later develop sustained hypertension
- There is some evidence that patients with white coat hypertension are closer to normotensive subjects than to mild hypotensive subjects in terms of target organ involvement
- Although they may not need blood pressure lowering drugs, general management, such as risk factor modifications, should be no different from that in patients requiring drug treatment
- An annual blood pressure measurement is advisable and, if conventional blood pressures show a tendency to rise, reassessment with 24 hour monitoring is indicated

Pregnancy—Twenty four hour ambulatory blood pressure measurement is being used increasingly in pregnancy where it has a number of indications. As in non-pregnant women, one of the major indications is identification of women with white coat hypertension. This condition, which occurs in about 10% of pregnant women, may lead to inaccurate diagnosis and management if not diagnosed. ABPM may also have a role in assessing the efficacy of antihypertensive treatment in pregnancy, and there are some indications that the technique may be a more sensitive predictor for the occurrence of pre-eclampsia than conventional measurement. Women who develop pre-eclampsia tend to lose the nocturnal dip in blood pressure but to date the sensitivity of this occurrence as a predictor for outcome has not been demonstrated in a longitudinal study.

As with the general population, studies have been performed in population samples to determine the normal reference values and characteristics of the 24 hour profile in pregnancy.

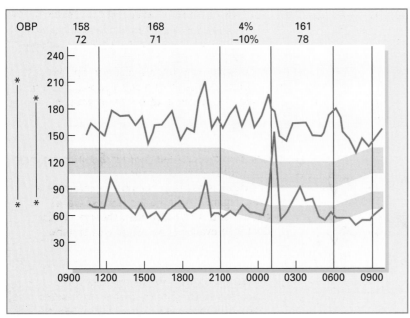

Plot of isolated hypertension: in this patient isolated systolic hypertension on OBP is sustained throughout the 24 hour period with a non-dipping nocturnal profile

Isolated systolic hypertension in elderly people—Elderly people are particularly susceptible to the adverse effects of antihypertensive drugs; those really needing drugs must be identified so that unnecessary treatment is avoided. A number of patients with isolated systolic hypertension do not have sustained elevation of pressure on ABPM and probably do not need treatment. ABPM allows identification of elderly patients with sustained elevation of systolic blood pressure and selection of those in need of treatment.

ABPM may prove particularly valuable in elderly people in whom blood pressure variability is increased (see also pages 14 and 15).

Nocturnal dipper status—There is growing evidence that subjects whose blood pressure does not decline at night — non-dippers — may be at higher risk than those who have a nocturnal fall in blood pressure — dippers. These hypertensive patients may be in need of careful blood pressure control and their identification is important. The only means of determining a patient's nocturnal dipping status is by ABPM.

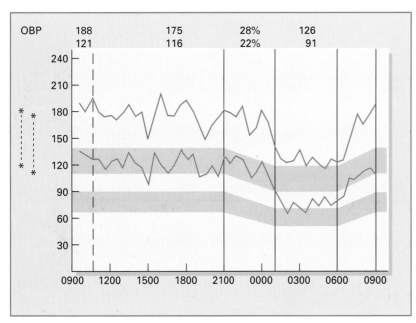

Plot of hypertension – a "dipper." Unlike the above plot, this patient with hypertension shows a nocturnal dip of 28/22%

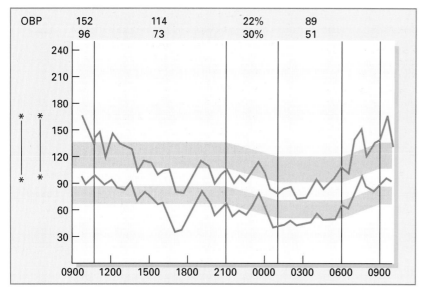

OBP	152		114		22%		89	
	96		73		30%		51	

Plot of hypotension: this elderly patient has elevated OBP which is carried into the ambulatory record for a short time and thereafter blood pressures are characterised by episodes of hypotension that were symptomatic

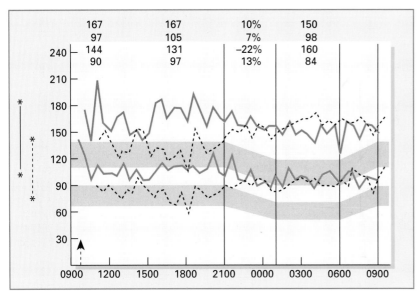

167		167		10%		150	
97		105		7%		98	
144		131		−22%		160	
90		97		13%		84	

In this patient the antihypertensive drug administered at 09:00 achieves day time but not night time control of blood pressure (unbroken line=before treatment, broken line=after treatment)

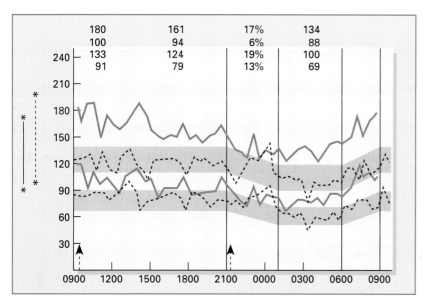

180		161		17%		134	
100		94		6%		88	
133		124		19%		100	
91		79		13%		69	

In this patient twice daily administration of a drug achieves 24 hour control of blood pressure

Evaluation of hypotensive symptoms—ABPM is proving useful in diagnosing symptoms resulting from low blood pressure, especially in elderly patients with autonomic failure. Whereas low blood pressure has been accepted as a cause of debility in mainland Europe, there has been a tendency to dismiss hypotension as of no consequence in the UK and the Republic of Ireland. ABPM is permitting a re-evaluation of this concept through the association of symptoms with the level of blood pressure.

Other diagnostic uses—Ambulatory measurement may also be helpful:

- In identifying episodic hypertension in phaeochromocytoma
- In characterising blood pressure behaviour in patients with secondary hypertension in whom the diurnal dipping pattern may be lost
- In diagnosing hypertension in special subgroups such as black people, children, elderly people, and pregnant women.

Selection and evaluation of antihypertensive drug treatment in clinical practice

ABPM is proving valuable in selecting a drug regimen suitable for the individual patient and it can also help the prescribing doctor to evaluate the efficacy of treatment.

Selection of drug and dosing regimen—Reference to the plot of 24 hour pressures enables the prescribing doctor to select the drug with a duration of action appropriate to the rise in pressure for that particular patient. There is some evidence that different groups of drugs may have different effects on the 24 hour blood pressure profile.

Efficacy of treatment—Efficacy of blood pressure control with antihypertensive drugs should be based on the 24 hour blood pressure profile rather than on sporadic measurements. ABPM can be particularly helpful in assessing drug efficacy in patients in whom office blood pressures indicate poor control — the resistant hypertensive.

Withdrawal of antihypertensive medication—Patients whose blood pressure was initially diagnosed by office measurement and whose blood pressure has been well controlled may merit a drug free period for reassessment with ABPM. Some of these patients may have white coat hypotension.

Patients in whom day time symptoms are troublesome can be evaluated with ABPM to determine if treatment is causing hypotension.

ABPM in studies of antihypertensive drug efficacy

- The ability of the technique to detect drug effects that may not be evident with conventional measurement
- Provision of information on the duration of antihypertensive drug effect
- Improvement of the design of studies of antihypertensive drug efficacy
- The ability of the technique to demonstrate the effect of drugs on nocturnal blood pressure
- Detection of the potential problems associated with excessive lowering of blood pressure
- Calculation of peak to trough ratio

- Some drugs may accentuate nocturnal dipping
- Others may blunt the normal nocturnal fall in blood pressure
- Others have no effect on diurnal rhythmicity

ABPM, although relatively new as a technique in clinical practice, is no stranger to hypertension research, where it has played an important part in the evaluation of antihypertensive drugs for many years.

In fact, the limitations of conventional measurement are such that serious consideration must be given to their place in studies of antihypertensive drug efficacy.

The advantages of ABPM over conventional techniques may be considered in relation to the factors in the box.

There is now evidence that hypertensive patients whose treated blood pressures are the lowest have the highest incidence of myocardial infarction. Attention must be directed not only to the efficacy of blood pressure reduction in studies of antihypertensive drugs but also to the magnitude of this reduction.

One of the most surprising aspects of research into this efficacy is the readiness with which a blood pressure lowering effect observed at one moment in the 24 hour cycle has been taken to indicate therapeutic efficacy for the whole day. With the increasing use of new formulations of drugs that permit once and twice daily dosage, it is now more important than ever to be able to assess the pattern as well as the duration of drug effect.

There is some evidence that different groups of antihypertensive drugs may perturb the circadian pattern of blood pressure in different ways. Hypertensive individuals on angiotensin converting enzyme inhibitors have been shown to have had markedly accentuated systolic and diastolic dipping patterns when compared with untreated hypertensives and patients on β blockers; however, hypertensive patients treated with β blockers, calcium antagonists, or diuretics had diastolic and systolic dipping patterns similar to those of the untreated groups. Whatever the explanation for these varying effects of different groups of antihypertensive drugs, the facts in the box raise important questions in assessing antihypertensive drug effects and in choosing a drug for an individual patient.

Acknowledgements

[1] O'Brien E, Murphy J, Tyndall A, Atkins N, Nee F, McCarthy G, Staessen J, Cox J, O'Malley K. Twenty-four-hour ambulatory blood pressure in men and women aged 17 to 80 years: the Allied Irish Bank Study. *J Hypertens* 1991;**9**:355–60.

Staessen J, Bulpitt CJ, Fagard R, Mancia G, O'Brien E, Thijs L, Vyncke G, Amery A. Reference values for the ambulatory blood pressure and the blood pressure measured at home: a population study. *J Human Hypertens* 1991;**5**:355–61.

Staessen J, Bulpitt CJ, O'Brien E, Cox J, Fagard R, Stanton A, Thijs L, Van Hulle S, Vyncke G, Amery A. The diurnal blood pressure profile: a population study. *Am J Hypertens* 1992;**5**:386–92.

Further reading

Bevan AT, Honour AJ, Stott FH. Direct arterial pressure recording in unrestricted man. *Clin Sci* 1969;**36**:329–44.

O'Brien E, Fitzgerald D, O'Malley K. Blood pressure measurement: current practice and future trends. *BMJ* 1985;**290**:729–34.

O'Brien, O'Malley K. Twenty-four hour ambulatory blood pressure measuring monitoring: a review of validation data. *J Hypertens* 1990;**8**(suppl 6):S11–16.

O'Brien E, Mee F, Atkins N, O'Malley K. Technical aspects of 24-hour ambulatory blood pressure monitoring: Comparative accuracy of six ambulatory systems determined by the BHS protocol. *High Blood Pressure* 1993;**2**(suppl 1):76–9.

O'Brien E, Atkins N, Mee F, O'Malley K. Comparative accuracy of six ambulatory devices according to blood pressure levels. *J Hypertens* 1993;**11**:673–5.

Cox J, O'Brien E, O'Malley K. Ambulatory blood pressure measurement in general practice. *Br J Gen Practice* 1992:402–3.

O'Brien E, Mee F, Atkins N, O'Malley K. Validation requirements for ambulatory blood pressure measuring systems. *J Hypertens* 1991;**9**(suppl 8):S13–15.

White WB, Lund-Johansen P, Omvik P. Assessment of four ambulatory blood pressure monitors and measurements by clinicians versus intrarterial blood pressure at rest and during exercise. *Am J Cardiol* 1990;**65**:60–6.

O'Brien E, Cox J, O'Malley K. The role of twenty-four-hour ambulatory blood pressure measurement in clinical practice. *J Hypertens* 1991;**9**(suppl 8):S63–5.

O'Brien E, Sheridan J, O'Malley K. Dippers and non-dippers. *Lancet* 1988;**ii**:397.

Pickering TG. The clinical significance of diurnal pressure variations: dippers and non-dippers. *Circulation* 1990;**81**:700.

Halligan A, O'Brien E, Walshe J, Darling M, O'Malley K. Clinical application of ambulatory blood pressure measurement in pregnancy. *J Hypertens* 1991;**9**(suppl 8):S75–7.

O'Brien E, O'Malley K. Ambulatory blood pressure monitoring in the evaluation of drug efficacy. *Am Heart J* 1991;**121**:999–1006.

O'Brien E, Cox J, O'Malley K. Ambulatory blood pressure measurement in the evaluation of blood pressure lowering drugs. *J Hypertens* 1989;**7**:243–7.

Waeber B, Scherrer U, Petrillo A, Bidiville J, Nussberger J, Waeber G, Hofstetter J-R, Brunner HR. Are some hypertensives overtreated? A prospective study of ambulatory blood pressure recording. *Lancet* 1987;**ii**:732–4.

PART II

BLOOD PRESSURE MANAGEMENT

D G BEEVERS
H J MARSHALL

HYPERTENSION AND CARDIOVASCULAR RISK

Definition of hypertension

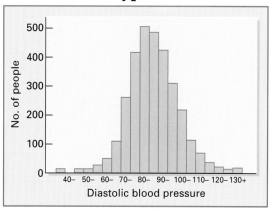

Diastolic blood pressure at screening in males in the Renfrew Study (1974). (From Hawthorne et al, 1974)

Blood pressure has a continuous (bell-shaped) distribution in the population. Consequently, there is no clear line separating normotensive from hypertensive patients. As the main concern of most clinicians regarding an individual's blood pressure is whether or not it requires treatment, the pragmatic definition of hypertension put forward by the late Professor Geoffrey Rose would seem to be the most universally acceptable:

"That level of blood pressure above which investigation and treatment do more good than harm."

This allows the physician some scope to take into account the patient's total cardiovascular risk as well as the evidence from published clinical trials of the usefulness of antihypertensive drugs in particular groups.

Risks of hypertension

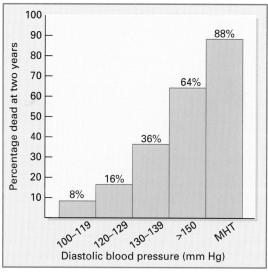

Severe hypertension in untreated patients. MHT, malignant hypertension. (From Leishman, 1959)

Leishman's original data on the mortality of patients with untreated severe hypertension alerted the medical profession to the enormous risks of a severely elevated blood pressure. Patients with diastolic blood pressures between 130 and 150 mm Hg with no retinopathy have only a 40% two year survival rate, the most common causes of death being stroke, myocardial infarction, heart failure, and renal failure. The introduction of drug treatment for hypertension meant that placebo controlled trials of severe hypertension became unethical. However, later population studies suggested that the close relationship between the height of the diastolic blood pressure and the risk of stroke and coronary heart disease extends into what could be regarded as the normotensive range.

Risk and diastolic blood pressure: (a) stroke and usual diastolic BP (in five categories defined by the baseline)—seven prospective observational studies and 843 events. (b) Coronary heart disease and usual diastolic BP (in five categories defined by the baseline)—nine prospective studies and 4856 events. (From MacMahon et al, 1990)

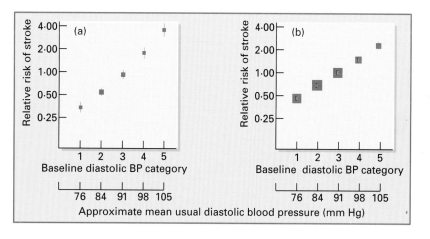

Hypertension and cardiovascular risk

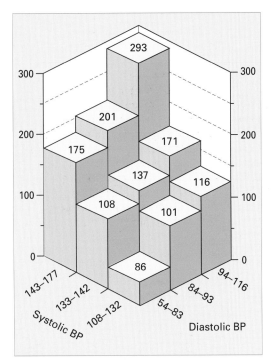

Ratio of actual to expected deaths from cardiovascular–renal disease. (From the Actuarial Society of America and the Association of Life Insurance Medical Directors, 1941)

These studies and their meta-analysis take no account of systolic blood pressure. However, contrary to popular belief, the height of the systolic blood pressure is a better predictor of cardiovascular risk than the diastolic pressure in patients over the age of 45 years. This has been shown from actuarial data and population surveys from America and, more recently, in clinical treatment trials where the benefits of treating isolated systolic hypertension have become apparent.

> **Over the age of 45, the height of the systolic blood pressure is a better predictor of risk than the diastolic pressure.**
> (The Framingham study)

Multiple risk factors

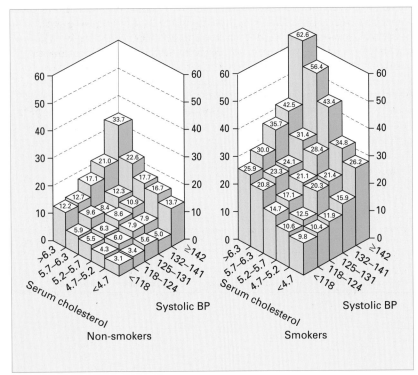

Coronary heart disease, mortality per 10 000 person-years (MRFIT). (From Stamler *et al*, 1986)

Individual risk

In assessing a patient's individual risk from hypertension, the other cardiovascular risk factors also need to be taken into consideration. Coexistent signs of end organ damage also confer a high degree of cardiovascular risk on a patient—for example, left venticular hypertrophy, previous heart attack, or stroke. However, these may indicate either severity or late detection of hypertension.

Smoking and hyperlipidaemia

The two most important independent risk factors that need to be taken into consideration are smoking and hyperlipidaemia. Data from the MRFIT trial show that these three risk factors have a synergistic effect. Thus a mildly hypertensive non-smoker with a normal serum cholesterol concentration is at much lower cardiovascular risk than a patient who also smokes and has a raised serum cholesterol concentration.

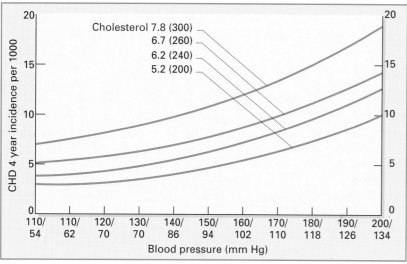

Coronary heart disease: four year incidence per 1000 in men aged 55 years. (From Stamler *et al*, 1986)

Age

Another factor to take into consideration when deciding about whether to treat hypertension must be the patient's age. Although the *relative risk* of cardiovascular mortality in a mildly hypertensive young man is raised, the *absolute risk* of sustaining a stroke or myocardial infarction within the next few years may well be low. However, for an elderly patient with the same degree of hypertension, the absolute risk of stroke or heart attack is much higher as the incidence of these conditions increases with age.

Multiple risk factors in hypertensive patients

Coexistent signs of end organ damage
Smoking and hyperlipidaemia
Age
Sex
Race
Public health/community risk factors

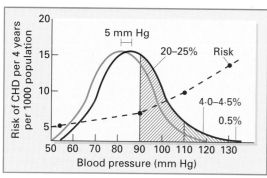

Blood pressure distribution: result of 5 mm Hg shift

Sex and race

Similarly, women, up to the age of about 50 years, have a lower risk for all levels of blood pressure than men. Ethnic differences may be important in calculating risk as hypertension and stroke are particularly common in black people and coronary artery disease is a major cause of death in people originating from the Indian subcontinent.

Community risk

In contrast to the strategy of assessing a patient's personal risk when making the decision to institute treatment, the public health approach to hypertension would suggest that we should consider community risk, based on the evidence that cardiovascular risk increases with diastolic blood pressure even within the normotensive range. It would seem appropriate to institute education programmes aimed at reducing the blood pressure of the community as a whole. By shifting the whole bell-shaped curve of blood pressure distribution 5 mm Hg to the left, there could be a reduction of community risk of stroke of about one third. Although it would still seem sensible to identify and treat high risk patients (that is, those with more severe hypertension), the community approach to blood pressure would probably be more cost effective: there are more normotensive and mildly hypertensive people in the population than severely hypertensive people; thus a reduction in the blood pressure of the whole population would reduce absolute numbers of strokes far more than focusing attention purely on those patients at high risk.

Further reading

Actuarial Society of America and the Association of Life Insurance Medical Directors. *Supplement to blood pressure study.* New York: Actuarial Society of America and the Association of Life Insurance Medical Directors, 1941.

Hawthorne VM, Greaves DA, Beevers DG. Blood pressure in a Scottish town. *BMJ* 1974;3:600–3.

Leishman AWD. Hypertension—treated and untreated: a study of 450 cases. *BMJ* 1959;1:1361.

MacMahon S, Peto R, Cutler J *et al*. Blood pressure, stroke and CHD, part 1. Prolonged differences in blood pressure: prospective observational studies collected for the regression dilution bias. *Lancet* 1990;335:765–74.

Stamler J, Wentworth D, Neaton JD, for the MRFIT Research Group. Relationship between serum cholesterol and risk of premature death from coronary heart disease: continuous and graded? Findings in 356 222 primary sciences of the Multiple Risk Factor Intervention Trial (MRFIT). *JAMA* 1986;256:2823–8.

BENEFITS OF BLOOD PRESSURE REDUCTION

The last 30 years has seen the introduction of a great many different classes of antihypertensive drugs, the newest agents having relatively few side effects. This means that millions of hypertensive patients can now have their blood pressure reduced, and the benefits of this reduction have been clearly demonstrated. Furthermore, new information has recently become available from the pooled results of all the randomised controlled trials that have been published over the years.

Severe hypertension

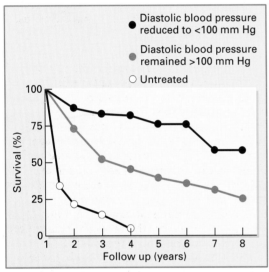

- ● Diastolic blood pressure reduced to <100 mm Hg
- ● Diastolic blood pressure remained >100 mm Hg
- ○ Untreated

Survival rates for untreated and treated malignant hypertension. (From Pickering, 1968)

Several non-controlled studies have been carried out of the treatment of malignant hypertension. The results of treatment were spectacular, with an 80% two year mortality being transformed with drugs to an 85% five year survival rate. Clinical trials of severe but non-malignant hypertension were published in the mid-1960s and again the results were impressive, with significant reductions in stroke and heart failure, but a rather disappointing impact on coronary heart disease.

Mild to moderate hypertension

Trial (or group of trials)	Numbers of events Treat:Control	Odds ratios and 95% confidence limits (Treat:Control)	
		TREATMENT BETTER ←	TREATMENT WORSE →
HDFP trial	102:158		
MRC 35–64 trial	60:109		
SHEP	105:162		
MRC 65–74 trial	101:134		
13 others	157:272		
All trials	525:835		38% (s.d. 4) reduction
(Heterogeneity $\chi_4^2 = 4\cdot2$ NS)			$2p < 0\cdot00001$

Reductions of stroke in the HDFP trial, SHEP trial, MRC trials, and in all 13 other smaller randomised trials of antihypertensive drug treatment. (From Collins and MacMahon, 1994)

The results of 16 unconfounded, randomised, controlled trials have been published since 1970. Some trials addressed the benefits of treating the higher grades of hypertension, five trials were exclusively conducted in older patients, and one concentrated on the benefits of treating isolated systolic hypertension. The four largest trials were the Hypertension Detection and Follow up Programme (HDFP) and the Systolic Hypertension in the Elderly Programme (SHEP) from the United States, and the two Medical Research Council (MRC) trials from Britain which examined separately the treatment of 35- to 64-year-old (MRC 35–64 trial) and 65- to 74-year-old (MRC 65–74 trial) patients respectively.

Preventing strokes
The benefits of reducing blood pressure in preventing strokes were impressive right from the start. The magnitude of the reduction of blood pressure achieved in the trials would be expected to bring about a 35–40% reduction in

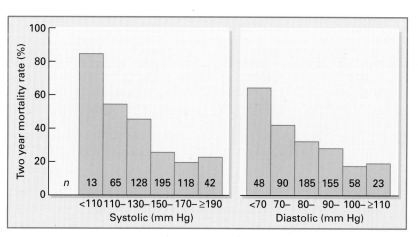

Trial (or group of trials)	Numbers of events Treat:Control	Odds ratios and 95% confidence limits (Treat:Control)	
		TREATMENT ← BETTER	TREATMENT WORSE →
HDFP trial	275:343		
MRC 35–64 trial	222:234		
SHEP	104:142		
MRC 65–74 trial	128:159		
13 others	205:226		
All trials	934:1104		16% (s.d. 4) reduction 2p = 0·00001
(Heterogeneity χ_4^2 = 4·3 NS)			

Reductions of coronary heart disease in the HDFP trial, SHEP trial, MRC trials, and in all 13 other smaller randomised trials of antihypertensive treatment. (From Collins and MacMahon, 1994)

Elderly hypertensive patients

Percentage change in cardiovascular events and overall death rate in elderly hypertensive patients in six randomised controlled trials

	Australian trial	EWPHE	Coope	SHEP	STOP-H	MRC
Strokes	−34	−36	−42	−36	−47	−25
Cardiac events	−19	−20	−15	−27	−13	−19
All deaths	−23	−9	−3	−13	−43	−3

EWPHE, European Working Party on Hypertension in the Elderly (from Amery *et al*, 1985).
Coope (from Coope and Warrender, 1986).
SHEP, Systolic Hypertension in the Elderly Programme (from SHEP, 1991).
STOP-H (from Dahlof *et al*, 1991).
MRC (from MRC Working Party, 1992).

Mortality rates of blood pressures in the very old (over 85 years) in Finland. (From Rajala *et al*, 1983)

strokes. The pooled trial data show that the actual reduction achieved was 38% (± 4%). This means that practically all strokes in hypertensive patients caused by their hypertension alone should be preventable. These benefits are apparent up to the age of about 80 years.

Preventing heart attacks

The results of the early trials conducted in younger patients had proved a little disappointing in their effects on coronary heart disease; in fact some smaller trials showed no benefits at all. However, the pooled data from all of the trials show a somewhat better picture mainly because of the excellent results in the more recent trials in older patients. Overall the expected reduction in heart attack was 20–25% and the pooled trial data show a 16% (± 4%) reduction which is highly significant and practically on target. It is interesting to note that much of this reduction was achieved with thiazide diuretic therapy, despite the adverse effects these drugs can have on plasma lipids.

Despite clear evidence of the benefits of treating hypertension in patients under 65 years of age, and the strong correlation between raised blood pressure and cardiovascular disease, there has traditionally been some reluctance to treat hypertension in older patients. This stemmed from a lack of large clinical trials particularly looking at elderly people and also the concept that elderly people may be a difficult group of patients to treat and that treatment may do more harm than good. However, the early 1990s have seen the publication of three large trials of antihypertensive treatment in elderly patients (SHEP, the Swedish Trial of Older Patients (STOP), and the MRC 64–75 trial). All the trials reported a reduction in mortality which reached significance in the STOP hypertension trial with a fall of 43%. Five of the six trials listed opposite showed significant reductions in total cardiovascular events and, as might have been expected, this was predominantly the result of a reduction in strokes. In those trials where side effects of drugs and metabolic disturbances were reported, they were all relatively minor. The message from these trials is that treatment of hypertension in the patients up to the age of 80 produces a reduction in mortality and morbidity.

In patients over 80 years of age, the trials were less convincing. There were some benefits apparent in this age group in the SHEP study, but the other trials did not support this unless there was severe systolic and diastolic hypertension. Observational data on blood pressure in very elderly people suggest that there may actually be an increased mortality with lower blood pressure, unless hypertension is severe, and this would concur with the findings of the STOP hypertension trial.

Systolic hypertension

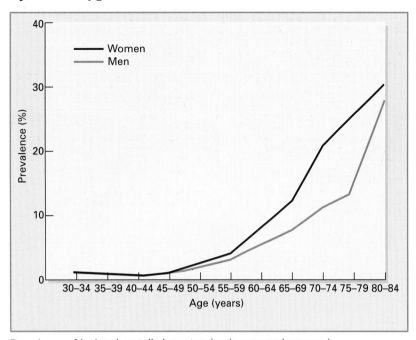

Prevalence of isolated systolic hypertension in men and women in Framingham, United States

Isolated systolic hypertension becomes more common with increasing age. Systolic blood pressure rises sharply with age and this may be the result of thickening of the brachial artery, and may thus reflect arterial damage. Even in the presence of a normal or low diastolic blood pressure, systolic hypertension remains an accurate predictor of cardiovascular risk. As a consequence, the treatment of isolated systolic hypertension would be expected to reduce cardiovascular risk.

Results of treating isolated systolic hypertension: the SHEP study

	Active treatment	Placebo
Total participants	2365	2371
Stroke	96	149
Transient ischaemic attack	62	82
Myocardial infarct	50	74
Coronary revascularisation needed	49	69
Left ventricular failure	48	102
Renal impairment	7	11
Total deaths	213	242

From SHEP (1991).

The SHEP study assessed the effect of treating isolated systolic hypertension (systolic blood pressure >160 mm Hg with diastolic blood pressure <90 mm Hg) in patients of 60 years and over with an average four years and 6 months follow up period. The treatment goal was to reduce systolic blood pressure to less than 160 mm Hg or by 20 mm Hg, whichever was the greater. This study showed a significant reduction in the incidence of stroke and a reduction in all cardiovascular events and mortality. This evidence is supported by subgroup analysis from the STOP hypertension trial and the MRC trial in elderly people.

Conclusions

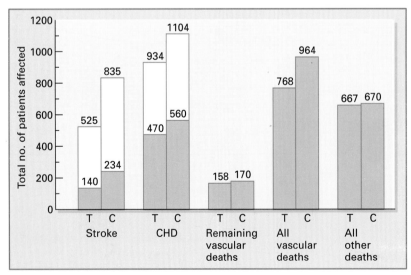

Meta-analysis of antihypertensive treatment: T, treated; C, control. ■ Fatal events; □ non-fatal events. (From Collins and MacMahon, 1994)

Antihypertensive treatment has now been shown to prevent heart attacks and strokes, and premature deaths. It could, therefore, be regarded as the most well validated, chronic, preventive, therapeutic manoeuvre. Further information is needed on the benefits of drug treatment in very old hypertensive patients and the optimum level to which blood pressure should be reduced. In addition, it is not yet known whether the newer antihypertensive drugs (that is, the angiotensin converting enzyme (ACE) inhibitors, the angiotensin receptor (AT1) antagonists, and the calcium channel blockers) will be as effective as the thiazides and the β blockers at preventing the vascular complications of hypertension. Trials comparing the different classes of antihypertensive therapy are currently under way.

Further reading

Amery A, Bakenhager W, Brixko P *et al*. Mortality and morbidity results from the European Working Party on High Blood Pressure in the Elderly Trial. *Lancet* 1985;i:1349.

Collins R, MacMahon S. Blood pressure, antihypertensive drug treatment and the risks of stroke and coronary heart disease. *Br Med Bull* 1994;**50**:272–98.

Coope J, Warrender TS. A randomised trial of hypertension in elderly patients in primary care. *BMJ* 1986;**293**:1145–52.

Dahlof B, Lindholm LH, Hanssen L, Shersten B, Ekbon T, Wester P-O. Morbidity and mortality in a Swedish trial of old patients with hypertension (STOP–hypertension). *Lancet* 1991;**338**:1281–4.

Hypertension Detection and Follow-up Programme Cooperative Group. The effect of treatment on mortality in "mild" hypertension. *N Engl J Med* 1982;**307**:976–80.

Medical Research Council Working Party. MRC trial of mild hypertension: principal results. *BMJ* 1985;**291**:97–104.

MRC Working Party. Medical Research Council Trial of treatment of hypertension in older adults: principal results. *BMJ* 1992;**304**:405–12.

Pickering G. *High blood pressure*. London: H & H Churchill, 1968.

Rajala S, Haavisto M, Heikinheimo R, Mattila K. Blood pressure and mortality in the very old (Letter). *Lancet* 1983;**ii**:520.

Systolic Hypertension in the Elderly Programme Cooperative Research Group. Prevention of stroke by antihypertensive drug treatment in older persons with isolated systolic hypertension. *JAMA* 1991;**265**:3255–64.

CAUSES OF HYPERTENSION

Epidemiology

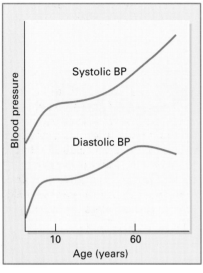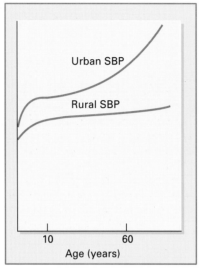

Blood pressure and age. Left: normal systolic (upper) and diastolic (lower) pressures in Westernised societies. Right: systolic blood pressure in urban societies (upper) and genetically similar tribal communities (lower) in Africa

Age
In Western societies systolic blood pressure rises with increasing age; diastolic blood pressure rises until the age of about 60 years, but thereafter tends to fall. However, in rural non-Westernised societies, hypertension is rare and the rise in pressure with age is minimal. Migration studies in Africa have, however, shown that members of rural tribes who migrate to urban areas develop a rapid rise in blood pressure within months of arrival. It would seem, therefore, that the rise in blood pressure with age is probably related mainly to socioeconomic and environmental factors.

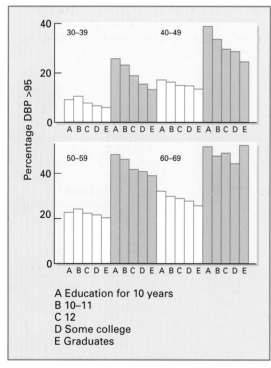

Prevalence of hypertension in black and white Americans in relation to duration of education. ■ Black Americans; □ white Americans. (From Hypertension Detection and Follow-up Program Cooperative Group, 1977)

Race
Most studies looking at blood pressure in black and white people in Western societies have shown a higher prevalence of hypertension in black people. This is in contrast to the picture in black people living in rural Africa, mentioned above. Even when correction is made—for obesity, socioeconomic, and dietary factors—there may still be some racially determined predisposition to hypertension. For example, plasma renin levels are generally lower in black compared with white people; as a result those drugs that antagonise the renin–angiotension system (β blockers and angiotensin converting enzyme inhibitors) are less effective. By contrast, people from the Indian subcontinent, who now live in Western countries, have similar blood pressure measurements to white people, although they have higher rates of coronary heart disease.

Migration studies on Japanese people moving from Japan to the west coast of America have shown that, when they lived in Japan, high blood pressure was common and stroke incidence high, although coronary heart disease was rare. On moving across the Pacific Ocean, there was a reduction in the incidence of hypertension and stroke, but a rise in the incidence of coronary heart disease.

These studies strongly suggest that, although there are racial differences in the predisposition to hypertension, environmental factors still play a significant role.

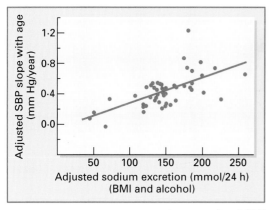

Intersalt project: data from 52 centres (*p*<0·001). SBP=systolic blood pressure; BMI=body mass index. (From Intersalt Cooperative Research Group, 1988)

Prevalence (%) of hypertension in underweight, normal, and overweight Americans

	At age	
Weight	20–39 years	40–69 years
Underweight	4·6	19·0
Normal	6·2	24·1
Overweight	14·9	37·1

Reproduced from Stamler *et al*, 1978.

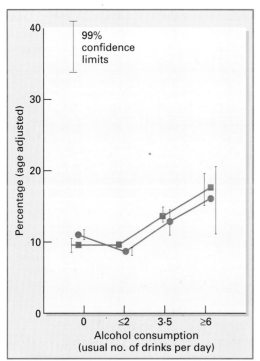

Prevalence of hypertension (diastolic blood pressure >95 mm Hg) in women (●) and men (■) in relation to usual alcohol consumption. (Reproduced with permission from Klatsky *et al*, 1977).

Salt ✓

There is now little doubt that salt intake has a direct effect on blood pressure. As stated earlier, migration studies in African and Japanese individuals have shown changes in blood pressure on moving from one environmental background to another, and the factor most likely to be involved in this change in blood pressure was a change in salt intake. The Intersalt project put the salt hypothesis beyond any reasonable doubt. Directly comparable data were obtained from 52 populations in 30 countries, when all the important confounding variables (in particular body mass and alcohol intake) were taken into account. The study showed quite clearly that the rise in blood pressure with advancing age in urban, but not rural, societies resulted from the amount of salt in the diet. This was supported by a recent meta-analysis of the many individual population surveys of blood pressure in relation to salt intake; it is further supported by a larger number of clinical trials which show reduction in blood pressure following salt restriction (see page 57).

Potassium ✓

The effect of dietary potassium intake on blood pressure is difficult to separate from that of salt. The Intersalt project did, however, show that high potassium intake was associated with a lower prevalence of hypertension. Studies looking at urinary sodium and potassium ratios in the United States showed marked differences between black and white people, although there was little difference in their sodium intake or excretion. As hypertension is more common in American black people this would support an independent role for potassium in lowering blood pressure. Clinical trials do show that an increase in potassium intake does have a modest antihypertensive effect.

Weight ✓

Fat people tend to have higher blood pressures than thin people. Even after taking into account the confounding effects of obese arms and inappropriate cuff sizes on blood pressure measurement, there is still a positive relationship between body mass index (BMI) and blood pressure. Clearly this association is related to an inceased caloric intake, although other dietary factors may also be implicated (for example, obese people may have a higher sodium intake). It has been postulated that obese people can have an increased tendency to exhibit insulin resistance and research is continuing into whether insulin resistance is involved in the pathogenesis of hypertension.

Alcohol ✓

Several epidemiological studies have shown a close positive relationship between alcohol consumption and blood pressure; the Intersalt study confirmed this trend. Overall, it would appear that the greater the alcohol consumption, the higher the blood pressure, although teetotallers appear to have slightly higher blood pressures than moderate drinkers. The reversibility of alcohol related hypertension has been shown in population surveys, and in alcohol loading and restriction studies. The mechanisms of the alcohol/blood pressure relationship are uncertain but they are not explained by body mass index or salt intake.

Causes of hypertension

Whilst there is good evidence that acute stressful stimuli do raise blood pressure, there is little convincing evidence that chronic stress causes hypertension.

Stress ✓

It has been suggested that psychological or environmental stress may play a part in the aetiology of hypertension. There is, however, little reliable evidence to support this. Studies of environmental stress levels in relation to hypertension have frequently been confounded by other environmental or lifestyle factors. Although stressful stimuli may cause an acute rise in blood pressure, it is still doubtful whether this has any significance in the long term. A reduction in psychological stress through biofeedback techniques may reduce blood pressure in the clinic; however, these techniques seem to have little effect on ambulatory home blood pressure recordings.

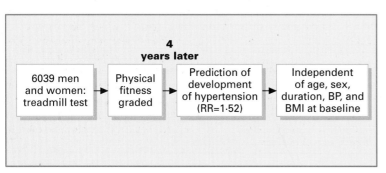

Epidemiological evidence that greater physical fitness protects against future hypertension. (From Blair *et al*, 1984)

Exercise

Blood pressure rises sharply during physical activity, although there is evidence that people who undertake regular exercise are fitter and healthier and have lower blood pressures. This may be because such people have a healthier diet and more sensible drinking and smoking habits. A recent study has, however, shown that there is an independent relationship between increased levels of exercise and lower blood pressures. The study suggests that vigorous exercise might be harmful, but all other grades of exercise are increasingly beneficial.

Pathophysiology of hypertension

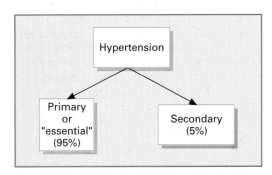

There is still much debate about the pathophysiology of hypertension. A small number of patients (between 2% and 5%) have an underlying renal or adrenal disease as the cause for their raised blood pressure. In the remainder, however, no clear identifiable cause is found and their condition is labelled "essential hypertension." A number of physiological mechanisms are involved in the maintenance of normal blood pressure and their derangement may play a part in the development of essential hypertension.

Physiological mechanisms involved in development of essential hypertension

Cardiac output
Peripheral resistance
Renin–angiotensin system
Autonomic nervous system
Other factors
    Bradykinin
    Endothelin
    EDRF (endothelial derived relaxing factor)
    ANP (atrial natriuretic peptide)
    Ouabain

Cardiac output and peripheral resistance

Maintenance of a normal blood pressure is dependent on the balance between cardiac output and peripheral resistance. Most patients with essential hypertension have a normal cardiac output but a raised peripheral vascular resistance. Peripheral resistance is determined not by large arteries or the capillaries but by small arterioles, the walls of which contain smooth muscle cells; contraction of smooth muscle cells is thought to be related to a rise in intracellular calcium concentration. This hypothesis is supported by the vasodilatory effect of drugs that block the calcium channel. Prolonged smooth muscle constriction is thought to induce structural changes with thickening of the arteriolar vessel walls; this provokes a further increase in arterial blood pressure.

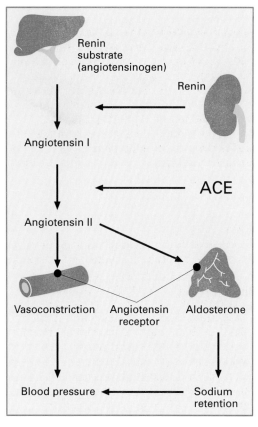

Renin–angiotensin system and effects on blood pressure and aldosterone release

Renin–angiotensin system

The renin–angiotensin system may be the most important of the hormonal systems that affect the control of blood pressure. Renin is secreted from the juxtaglomerular apparatus of the kidney in response to glomerular underperfusion or a reduced salt intake. It is also released in response to stimulation from the sympathetic nervous system. Renin is responsible for converting renin substrate to angiotensin I, a physiologically inactive substance which is converted to angiotensin II by angiotensin converting enzyme (ACE). Angiotensin II is a potent vasoconstrictor and thus causes a rise in blood pressure. In addition it stimulates the release of aldosterone from the zona glomerulosa of the adrenal gland, which results in a further rise in blood pressure related to sodium retention. The circulating renin–angiotensin system is not thought to be directly responsible for the rise in blood pressure in essential hypertension. In particular, many hypertensive patients have low levels of renin and angiotensin II (especially elderly and black people), and drugs that block the renin system are not particularly effective in these people. There is, however, increasing evidence that there are important non-circulating "local" renin–angiotensin systems that do control blood pressure—for example, there are local renin systems in the kidney and the arterial tree which have important roles in regulating blood flow.

Autonomic nervous system

Sympathetic nervous system stimulation can cause both arteriolar constriction and ateriolar dilatation. Thus the autonomic nervous system has an important role in maintaining a normal blood pressure. It is also important in the mediation of short term changes in blood pressure in response to stress and physical exercise. There is, however, little evidence to suggest that adrenaline and noradrenaline have any clear role in the aetiology of hypertension. Nevertheless, their effects are important, not least because drugs that block the sympathetic nervous system do lower blood pressure and have a well established therapeutic role. It is probable that hypertension is related to an interaction between the autonomic nervous system and the renin–angiotensin system, together with other factors, including sodium, circulating volume, and some of the more recently described hormones discussed below.

Other factors affecting blood pressure control

There are many other vasoactive systems and mechanisms affecting sodium transport and vascular tone that are involved in the maintenance of a normal blood pressure. It is not clear, however, what part these play in the development of essential hypertension. Bradykinin is a potent vasodilator which is inactivated by angiotensin converting enzyme. Consequently, the angiotensin converting enzyme inhibitors may exert some of their effect through actions on this system. Endothelin is a recently discovered, powerful, vascular, endothelial vasoconstrictor which may produce a salt sensitive rise in blood

The autonomic nervous system and its control of blood pressure. (Adapted from Swales *et al*, 1991)

Causes of hypertension

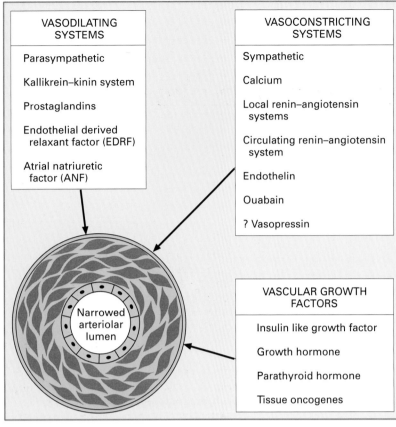

VASODILATING SYSTEMS

Parasympathetic

Kallikrein–kinin system

Prostaglandins

Endothelial derived relaxant factor (EDRF)

Atrial natriuretic factor (ANF)

VASOCONSTRICTING SYSTEMS

Sympathetic

Calcium

Local renin–angiotensin systems

Circulating renin–angiotensin system

Endothelin

Ouabain

? Vasopressin

Narrowed arteriolar lumen

VASCULAR GROWTH FACTORS

Insulin like growth factor

Growth hormone

Parathyroid hormone

Tissue oncogenes

The control of peripheral arteriolar resistance. (Adapted from Swales *et al*, 1991)

pressure. It also activates local renin–angiotensin systems. Endothelial derived relaxant factor (EDRF) is produced by arterial and venous endothelium and diffuses through the vessel wall into the smooth muscle causing vasodilatation.

Atrial natriuretic peptide (ANP) is a recently described hormone secreted from atria of the heart in response to increased blood volume. Its effect is to increase sodium excretion from the kidney. A defect in this system may cause fluid retention and hypertension. Sodium transport in vasular smooth muscle is also thought to influence blood pressure via its interrelationship with calcium transport across cell membranes. Ouabain is also a naturally occurring substance which is thought to interfere with cell sodium and calcium transport, giving rise to vasoconstriction.

Further reading

Blair SN, Goodyear NN, Gibbons WW, Cooper KH. Physical fitness and incidence of hypertension in healthy normotensive men and women. *JAMA* 1984;252:487–90.

Intersalt Cooperative Research Group. Intersalt: an international study of electrolyte excretion and blood pressure. Results for 24 hour urinary sodium and potassium excretion. *BMJ* 1988;297:319–28.

Klatsky AL, Friedman GD, Siegelaub AB, Gerard MD. Alcohol consumption and blood pressure, Kaiser Permanente Multiphasic Health Examination Data. *N Engl J Med* 1977;296:1194–200.

Stamler R, Stamler J, Riedlinger WF *et al.* Weight and blood pressure: findings in hypertension screening of 1 million Americans. *JAMA* 1978;240:1607–10.

Hypertension Detection and Follow-up Program Cooperative Group. Race, education and prevalence of hypertension. *Am J Epidemiol* 1977;106:351–61.

Swales JD, Sever PS, Peart WS. *Clinical atlas of hypertension.* London: Gower Medical, 1991.

PATIENT ASSESSMENT I: CLINICAL

History

Symptoms

In the absence of any other illness or the complications of hypertension, most newly diagnosed hypertensive patients have no specific symptoms. This is reflected in the fact that many are diagnosed as an incidental finding at a routine medical examination or attendance at the doctor for some other condition. There has been a common misconception that hypertensive patients complain of headaches, epistaxis, and lethargy. Although occasionally headache may be encountered, in fact, even severely hypertensive individuals often have no symptoms until they present with a heart attack or a stroke. Hypertension has justly been described as the "silent killer." When taking a history, therefore, it is important to inquire specifically about symptoms relating to the complications of hypertension or conditions that may affect the management of the patient's blood pressure or the choice of drugs.

Medical history

This may well give clues to the presence of the causes or complications of hypertension. For women, it is particularly important to inquire into their obstetric history particularly about pre-eclampsia or pregnancy related hypertension.

Family history

A family history of hypertension is found in many patients who themselves have essential hypertension. It is important to elicit whether there is strong family history of ischaemic heart disease, stroke, or premature cardiovascular death because this has a strong influence on the patient's own risk of cardiovascular disease. A family history of diabetes should alert the clinician to the possibility that the patient may also be diabetic. It is also important to exclude any family history of renal disease which may cause hypertension—for example, autosomal dominant polcystic kidney disease.

Drug history

It is obviously necessary to ascertain whether the patient is already taking antihypertensive medication and whether there has been past intolerance to any drugs. It is also important to establish whether the

Drugs affecting blood pressure

- Drugs causing sodium retention: oral corticosteroids, ACTH, liquorice, carbenoxolone, phenylbutazone, indomethacin
- Drugs causing increased sympathomimetic activity: ephedrine, cold cures, monoamine oxidase inhibitors
- Direct vasoconstrictors: ergot alkaloids
- Oral contraceptives, oestrogen therapy
- Drug withdrawal: clonidine
- Interactions with antihypertensive drugs: tricyclic antidepressants, indomethacin

patient is taking any treatment that would either cause or exacerbate hypertension (for example, the oral contraceptive pill or carbenoxolone) or any medication that might interact with antihypertensive drugs (for example, non-steroidal anti-inflammatory drugs which may inhibit the effects of angiotensin converting enzyme inhibitors).

Social history

The main object of a social history in the context of hypertension is to assess the patient's risk factors for both hypertension and cardiovascular disease in general. Thus it is necessary to inquire about the patient's alcohol intake, dietary habits including salt and fat consumption, and, most important of all, whether or not the patient smokes tobacco.

Physical examination

Features suggestive of acromegaly

Early
- Amenorrhoea
- Impotence
- Deep voice
- Increase in size of hands/feet
- Coarsened facial features

Late
- Visual disturbance
- Headache
- Characteristic appearance
- Glucose intolerance
- Depression

General

One of the most important aspects of the examination of any hypertensive patient is the measurement of height and weight. These can be used to calculate the body mass index which will allow a more accurate measure of obesity. Body weight should be checked at all subsequent consultations.

$$\text{Body mass index} = \frac{\text{Weight (kg)}}{[\text{Height (m)}]^2}$$

$\text{BMI} \geqslant 30 = \text{obese}$
$\text{BMI} = 25\text{--}29 = \text{overweight}$
$\text{BMI} < 25 = \text{normal}$

As with the clinical history, physical examination should include a search for the causes and the effects of hypertension, and evidence of other cardiovascular risk factors and diseases that may affect the choice of management.

General examination may reveal the distinctive appearance of acromegaly or Cushing's syndrome, xanthelasmata associated with hyperlipidaemia, or nicotine staining of the fingers. The last is an important physical sign in heavy smokers.

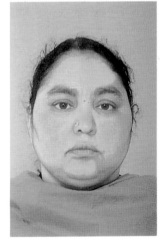

Patient with Cushing's disease and hypertension (reproduced with permission of the patient)

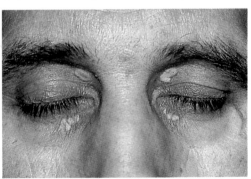

Bilateral xanthelasmata in a hypertensive patient

Cardiovascular

Cardiovascular examination may reveal absent pulses or arterial bruits reflecting atheromatous disease in the femoral or carotid arteries. There may be evidence of left ventricular hypertrophy on examination of the heart, and auscultation may reveal a loud aortic second sound. A loud systolic murmur across the chest and back, in association with delayed femoral pulses and a blood pressure differential between the arms and legs, may result from a coarctation of the aorta. A high pitched early diastolic murmur suggests aortic regurgitation which could give rise to a wide pulse pressure and apparent isolated systolic hypertension.

Chest

Examination of the chest may give evidence of obstructive airway disease which would mean avoiding the use of β blockers. Pulmonary crepitations may be an indication of heart failure.

Physical examination

- General
- Cardiovascular system
- Chest
- Abdomen
- Central nervous system
- Eyes

Abdominal

Examination of the abdomen may reveal signs of chronic liver disease associated with high alcohol ingestion. Polycystic kidneys may also be palpable on abdominal examination and a vascular bruit audible lateral to the midline might suggest renal artery stenosis. (Almost 50% of patients with severe hypertension and peripheral vascular disease have renal artery stenosis on renal angiography.)

Central nervous system

Central nervous system examination may reveal evidence of old stroke disease. Neuropsychiatric assessment may indicate the presence of multi-infarct dementia.

Retinal changes associated with hypertension

Mild
   Vessel tortuosity
   Silver wiring
   Arteriovenous nipping
Severe
   Flame shaped retinal haemorrhages
   Hard exudates (macular star)
   Cotton wool spots
   Papilloedema

Examination of the eyes   eyes & kidney

Ophthalmoscopy is obligatory for all patients with moderate to severe hypertension. The retinal changes can be mild or severe. The appearance of features associated with more severe hypertensive retinopathy coincides with the development of fibrinoid necrosis in the arterioles of the kidney and many other organs—a feature of the syndrome of malignant hypertension; if left untreated this is associated with a 80% two year mortality rate.

Ophthalmoscopy may also reveal changes suggestive of diabetic retinopathy or the characteristic appearances of retinal vein or artery occlusion which are more common in hypertensive patients.

Further reading

Hart JT. *Hypertension, community control of high blood pressure*, 3rd edn. Oxford: Radcliffe Medical Press, 1993.

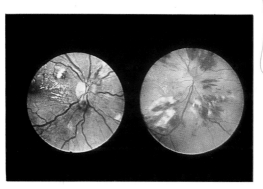

Cotton wool spots in malignant hypertension

PATIENT ASSESSMENT II: INVESTIGATIONS

Investigations for all hypertensive patients

- Urinalysis
- Biochemistry
  - —Serum sodium
  - —Serum potassium
  - —Serum urea and creatinine
  - —Serum calcium
  - —Serum uric acid
  - —Serum lipid levels
  - —γ-Glutamyl transferase
- Haematology
- Electrocardiography

Tests used for the investigation of hypertensive patients can be divided into those that should be done in all newly diagnosed hypertensives and those that should be reserved for certain patients in whom the likelihood of finding a specific cause is particularly high. More detailed investigation is necessary in patients under the age of 40 years, those with resistant hypertension (that is, not responding to a combination of two or more drugs), those with severe hypertension (diastolic blood pressure > 120 mm Hg), and those in whom clinical assessment or baseline investigations suggest that there may be an underlying cause of secondary hypertension. Investigations are also aimed at detecting hypertensive end organ damage which when present is a potent predictor of an individual's risk of death.

Investigations for all hypertensive patients

The tests outlined below should be done in all patients within the primary and secondary health care setting.

Urinalysis

Routine stick testing of urine is the simplest but often the most revealing of the basic investigations of hypertension. Proteinuria and microscopic haematuria may both result from renal arteriolar necrosis in patients with malignant hypertension and occur in patients with non-malignant hypertension and hypertensive nephrosclerosis. They may also indicate intrinsic renal disease such as glomerulonephritis (particularly IgA nephropathy), polycystic kidney disease, or chronic pyelonephritis. Haematuria can also occur in urological malignancy, and glycosuria may indicate coincident diabetes mellitus.

In those cases where proteinuria is present, for a given level of blood pressure, the risk of death is roughly doubled.

A benign adrenal adenoma taken from a patient with Conn's syndrome (primary hyperaldosteronism)

Biochemical investigations

Serum sodium concentration—This may be raised or be in the high normal range in patients with primary hyperaldosteronism (Conn's syndrome). In contrast, in patients with secondary hyperaldosteronism, as occurs in chronic renal failure, serum sodium concentration can be low or low/normal. Another cause of a low serum sodium concentration is the use of high doses of diuretics, where occasionally profound hyponatraemia may be encountered.

A serum potassium concentration of less than 3·5 mmol/l should be rechecked. If potassium concentration is persistently low, aldosterone excess should be considered.

Serum potassium concentration—This is usually low in patients with Conn's syndrome, although it may also be low in patients receiving diuretic therapy. These drugs need to be stopped for several weeks before a true baseline serum potassium can be established. Hyperkalaemia may be found in renal failure or with the use of some antihypertensive drugs such as angiotensin converting enzyme (ACE) inhibitors or potassium sparing diuretics (for example, spironolactone or amiloride). ACE inhibitors and potassium sparing diuretics should never be used together.

Serum urea and creatinine concentrations—Hypertension may cause renal impairment and renal diseases cause hypertension; serum creatinine levels therefore need regular monitoring. A graph plotting the reciprocal of the serum creatinine against time may give an indication of the rate of deterioration of renal function, and hence predict the need for intervention and renal replacement therapy. Hypertensive patients with even a modest increase in serum creatinine need more detailed investigation, usually in a hospital clinic.

Serum calcium concentration—Chronic renal failure may cause a low serum calcium with a raised serum phosphate concentration. By contrast, primary hyperparathyroidism, which may be associated with hypertension, causes a raised serum calcium with a low serum phosphate concentration. As with serum potassium, however, these results may be affected by the use of diuretic therapy, so these need to be stopped before true baseline levels can be established.

Serum uric acid concentration—Hyperuricaemia is found in about 40% of hypertensive patients, in particular when there is renal impairment. There is also an elevation of serum uric acid with either increased alcohol ingestion or the use of thiazide diuretics.

Serum lipid concentrations—Although not directly related, elevated serum cholesterol and triglyceride levels with low HDL cholesterol are synergistic risk factors which need to be assessed and treated if necessary. They may also be elevated slightly by the use of some antihypertensive agents, for example, thiazide diuretics and β blockers.

γ-Glutamyl transferase levels—Raised γ-glutamyl transferase levels strongly suggest a raised alcohol intake, assuming that other intrinsic liver diseases have been excluded. There are strong associations between alcohol abuse and hypertension.

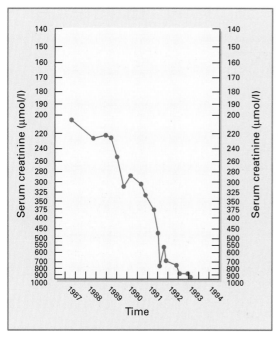

Example of a reciprocal creatinine chart in a patient with chronic renal failure

Haematological findings

Abnormality	Possible significance
Normochromic/normocytic anaemia	Chronic renal failure
	Underlying connective tissue disease
Raised mean cell volume	High alcohol intake
Leucopenia	Use of certain drugs—for example, methyldopa
Low platelet count	Underlying connective tissue disease
Polycythaemia	Renal carcinoma
	Obstructive airway disease

Haematology

Although a full blood count is a simple test, it is unlikely to provide a clear pointer to the cause or effects of hypertension. Polycythaemia may, however, result from a renal carcinoma or, more commonly, from either obstructive airway disease or high alcohol ingestion.

Electrocardiography

This should be a routine investigation on all newly diagnosed hypertensive patients, as it provides a baseline with which later changes may be compared. In addition, it may show evidence of underlying ischaemic heart disease. The most important feature of the ECG in hypertension is, however, left ventricular hypertrophy (LVH) which provides clear evidence of end organ damage and a three- to fourfold excess mortality; it also indicates the need for good blood pressure control. Left ventricular hypertrophy is diagnosed when the sum of the S wave in lead V1 or V2 and the R wave in lead V5 or V6 is 35 mm or more. The prognosis is even worse if the "strain" pattern is present (ST depression and/or T wave inversion in leads V5 and V6).

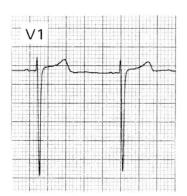
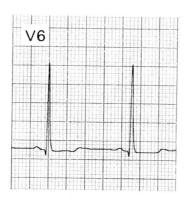

ECGs demonstrating left ventricular hypertrophy and strain

Investigations for selected patients

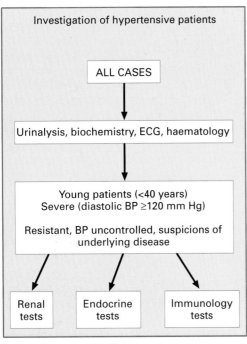

Investigation of hypertensive patients

ALL CASES

↓

Urinalysis, biochemistry, ECG, haematology

↓

Young patients (<40 years)
Severe (diastolic BP ≥120 mm Hg)

Resistant, BP uncontrolled, suspicions of underlying disease

↓

| Renal tests | Endocrine tests | Immunology tests |

Criteria for more detailed investigations

More detailed investigation is only necessary in a small minority of patients, and most commonly it is necessary to refer such patients to specialised centres.

Twenty four hour urine collection

A careful 24 hour urine collection can provide valuable information in the further investigation of hypertensive patients.

- A measurement of 24 hour urinary sodium excretion may give some indication of the patient's sodium intake and provide a basis for counselling. Patient's 24 hour sodium intake should be reduced to around 100 mmol/l.
- For those patients whose urinalysis shows proteinuria, the 24 hour urine collection allows accurate quantification; those with more than 1 g proteinuria per 24 hours may require more specialised tests, including a renal biopsy and immunology. NB In diabetic patients microalbuminuria (< 300 mg/24 hours) indicates early diabetic nephropathy.
- In those patients with a history suggestive of the diagnosis of phaeochromocytoma—that is, paroxysmal or severe hypertension with sweating and palpitations, the 24 hour urine collection will allow measurement of catecholamine metabolites such as metanephrines or vanillyl mandelic acid (VMA).
- Cases of suspected Cushing's syndrome are investigated with an assessment of 24 hour urinary free cortisol, in addition to plasma cortisol profiles.
- Estimation of creatinine clearance is not necessary unless there is severe renal failure.

Radiology

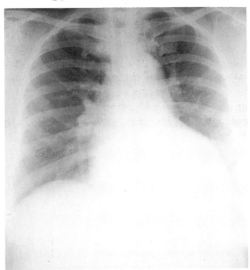

Chest radiograph of patient with malignant hypertension, showing cardiomegaly

Chest radiography

A chest radiograph is not necessary in most hypertensive patients. It is, however, indicated when there is evidence of cardiac or respiratory disease. It is best to ask the radiologist specifically to report the cardiothoracic ratio as this will provide a crude measure of the amount of left ventricular hypertrophy.

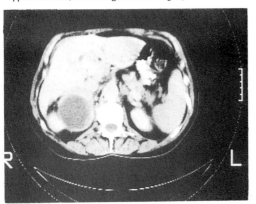

CT scan of phaeochromocytoma

Computed tomography

This is now the investigation of choice for the localisation of phaeochromocytomas or adrenal tumours causing aldosterone excess. Small tumours may, however, still be missed and computed tomography may not pick up generalised adrenal hyperplasia.

Renal imaging

Ultrasonography is the renal imaging procedure of first choice in hypertensive patients. Renal ultrasonography or intravenous urography are useful in demonstrating renal anatomy when urinalysis or serum biochemistry suggests a diagnosis of renal disease. Either technique can demonstrate hydronephrosis, polycycstic kidneys, or diminished renal size. A unilateral, smooth, small kidney may indicate renal artery stenosis that requires further investigation. Intravenous urography is then worthwhile and may show a delay in renal opacification on one side with later paradoxical hyperconcentration. Abdominal ultrasound may also show adrenal tumours in thin people.

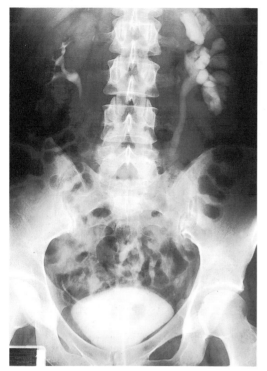

Intravenous urogram showing left hydronephrosis

Renal angiography

This is the gold standard for the diagnosis of renal artery stenosis, although the procedure does carry some risk; and should be reserved for specialist investigation. It may be indicated in patients with severe resistant hypertension even when other evidence of renal artery stenosis is lacking. Renal artery stenosis due to fibromuscular hyperplasia in young people may be curable by angioplasty.

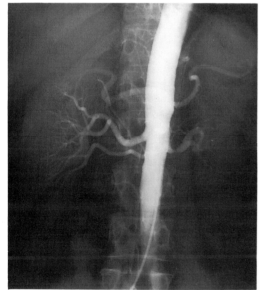

Radioisotope imaging

Standard renal radioisotope imaging now has little to offer in the investigation of hypertension. The captopril renogram may, however, give additional evidence in support of the diagnosis of renal artery stenosis. In this test, radioisotope imaging of the kidneys is performed before and after administration of a dose of captopril. The isotope image of the kidney on the affected side is reduced following the captopril dose. Radioisotope imaging may also be useful in the localisation of phaeochromocytomas using scans with ^{131}I-labelled *meta*-iodobenzylguanidine (MIBG scan).

Left renal artery stenosis on a renal arteriogram

Echocardiography

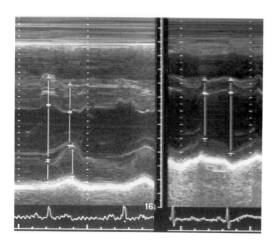

This is primarily of use in the investigation of cardiac murmurs discovered on routine examination, although echocardiography does in fact provide the gold standard for the measurement of left ventricular hypertrophy. At present, it remains impractical to perform echocardiography on all hypertensive patients and a diagnosis of left ventricular hypertrophy (LVH) is usually on the basis of the ECG or the chest radiograph.

M-mode echocardiograms showing: left: severe left ventricular hypertrophy with marked thickening of the intraventricular septum and posterior wall; right: normal echocardiogram

Plasma hormone concentrations

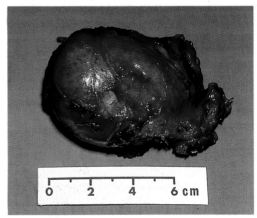

Phaeochromocytoma removed from a patient with Sipple's syndrome

These may be useful in confirming the diagnosis of an endocrine cause of secondary hypertension. Conn's syndrome results in raised plasma aldosterone concentrations with suppressed plasma renin activity. In contrast, secondary hyperaldosteronism gives rise to raised plasma aldosterone concentrations together with raised plasma renin activity. It is important that these tests are measured with the patient both fasting and supine, preferably before rising in the morning.

The investigation of Cushing's syndrome may involve measuring plasma cortisol and ACTH concentrations. Twenty four hour plasma cortisol profiles may be required to elicit the diagnosis. The differentiation between ACTH secreting tumours and adrenal tumours secreting cortisol requires specialised endocrinological tests and computed tomography scans.

Acromegaly may be suspected from the clinical appearance of the patient; its investigation is through glucose tolerance testing with plasma growth hormone levels and computed tomography scans of the pituitary fossa.

Primary hyperparathyroidism is diagnosed by the presence of a normal or raised parathyroid hormone concentration in the presence of raised serum calcium concentration. The diagnosis of phaeochromocytoma is normally made from a combination of the patient's symptoms and the 24 hour urinary catecholamine analysis. This technique will, however, miss the diagnosis in a few patients and plasma noradrenaline concentrations may then be useful in those patients in whom there is a high index of suspicion.

Further reading
Beevers DG, MacGregor BA. *Hypertension in practice*, 2nd edn. London: Dunitz, 1995.

TREATMENT OF UNCOMPLICATED HYPERTENSION

Non-pharmacological treatment

Correctable lifestyle factors for hypertension

- Obesity
- Salt
- Alcohol
- Exercise

The evidence in the chapter on causes of hypertension suggests that there are factors in the lifestyle of may hypertensive patients that can be modified to produce a reduction in blood pressure. Many reliable studies now confirm that weight reduction, restriction of salt intake, and moderation of alcohol intake, as well as increased exercise, can produce beneficial effects on blood pressure. These may obviate the need for pharmacological treatment or at least have an additive effect when combined with drug therapy. In some patients, stringent non-pharmacological measures may even allow reduction in or cessation of drug therapy. The current guidelines of the British Hypertension Society (see Sever, 1993) and the US Joint National Committee urge that non-pharmacological measures should be used in all hypertensive patients.

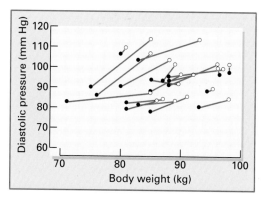

Diastolic pressure before (○) and after (●) body weight reduction: overview analysis. (Reproduced from Staessen et al, 1988)

Obesity

There is a strong association between obesity and hypertension. Several studies have shown that a reduction in systolic and diastolic pressures occurs with weight loss: a reduction in weight of 3 kg produces an estimated fall in blood pressure of 7/4 mm Hg; one of 12 kg gives a fall of 21/13 mm Hg. Every attempt should be made to encourage obese patients to diet so that their weight falls to within the norm for their height and build. Available evidence suggests that the results achieved with the help of dietitians are better than those achieved by medical staff alone.

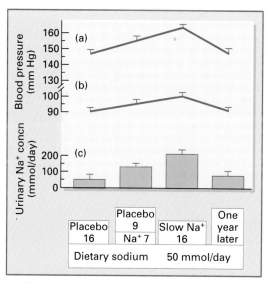

Effects on (a) systolic blood pressure, (b) diastolic blood pressure, and (c) urinary sodium restriction of giving three levels of supplementation to sodium restricted patients. (From MacGregor et al, 1989)

Salt

As suggested by the Intersalt study, there is a clear relationship between dietary salt intake and blood pressure. Salt restriction to about 100 mmol/day has been shown to produce a significant reduction in blood pressure in several randomised placebo controlled studies. Suitable dietary salt restriction can be achieved by not adding salt at the dining table and avoiding notoriously salty foods such as hamburgrs, sausages, and salty bacon. This may produce a reduction in blood pressure similar to that seen with the use of diuretics and, of course, it carries fewer side effects.

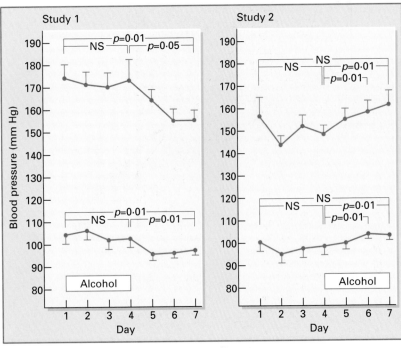

The effects of alcohol or abstinence on systolic and diastolic blood pressures. (From Potter and Beevers, 1984)

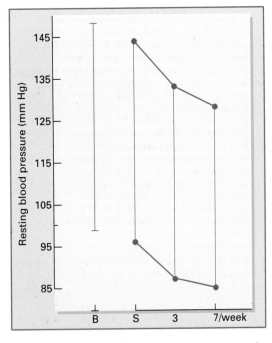

Resting supine blood pressure at three levels of physical activity: baseline measurement (B), sedentary activity (S), three times/week exercise (3), and seven times/week exercise (7). (From Nelson *et al*, 1986)

Alcohol

As mentioned in the chapter on causes of hypertension (page 45), the association between alcohol intake and hypertension is well documented in both population and clinical studies. An alcohol intake of around 80 g alcohol/day (equivalent to 4 pints of beer) has been shown to raise blood pressure, particularly in hypertensive patients. Blood pressure falls soon after drinking is stopped or reduced and remains low in those who continue to abstain. Where relevant, hypertensive patients should be encouraged to reduce their alcohol intake to an average of 21 units/week in men and 14 units/week in women (1 unit being equivalent to one glass of wine or sherry, one tot of spirits, or half a pint of beer).

Exercise

Epidemiological studies on exercise and blood pressure are difficult to assess because they can easily be counfounded by differences in diet and lifestyle. There are, however, some reliable studies now available which show that a graduated exercise programme is associated with clinically useful reductions in blood pressure in hypertensive patients. Newly diagnosed, obese, hypertensive patients with ischaemic heart disease should not suddenly take up jogging, but a sensibly administered increase in physical exercise is beneficial in such patients.

When to use drugs?

As mentioned previously, the most pragmatic definition of hypertension is: "That level of blood pressure above which investigation and treatment do more good than harm" (Grimley Evans and Rose, 1971).

With this in mind, guidelines for treatment have been devised taking into consideration the available data on the risks of hypertension and the benefits of its treatment. The current British and American guidelines suggest that we should use drug treatment in those patients

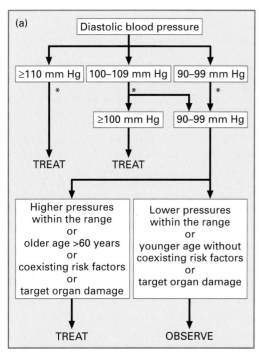

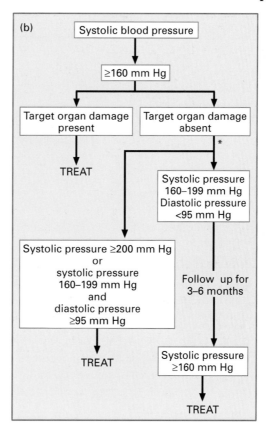

(a)

Diastolic blood pressure

≥110 mm Hg | 100–109 mm Hg | 90–99 mm Hg

≥100 mm Hg | 90–99 mm Hg

TREAT | TREAT

Higher pressures within the range or older age >60 years or coexisting risk factors or target organ damage

Lower pressures within the range or younger age without coexisting risk factors or target organ damage

TREAT | OBSERVE

(b)

Systolic blood pressure

≥160 mm Hg

Target organ damage present | Target organ damage absent

TREAT

Systolic pressure 160–199 mm Hg Diastolic pressure <95 mm Hg

Systolic pressure ≥200 mm Hg or systolic pressure 160–199 mm Hg and diastolic pressure ≥95 mm Hg

Follow up for 3–6 months

TREAT

Systolic pressure ≥160 mm Hg

TREAT

Thresholds for drug treatment of hypertension with reference to (a) diastolic blood pressure and (b) systolic blood pressure >160 mm Hg. (All patients given non-pharmacological advice.) *Repeat measurements. (Taken from the British Hypertension Guidelines, in Sever et al, 1993)

Which drugs to use?

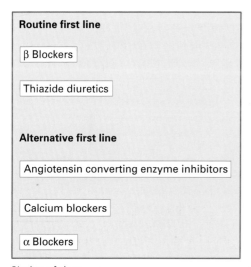

Routine first line

β Blockers

Thiazide diuretics

Alternative first line

Angiotensin converting enzyme inhibitors

Calcium blockers

α Blockers

Choice of drug

under 80 years of age with a diastolic blood pressure of ≥ 100 mm Hg and between 90 and 99 mm Hg when there is evidence of end organ damage or coexisting risk factors. In addition, they recommend that we should treat patients (particularly those aged over 60) with systolic blood pressures ≥ 160 mm Hg even if the diastolic blood pressures are lower than 90 mm Hg. The guidelines also urge that blood pressures should be measured on four separate occasions before taking the decision to prescribe antihypertensive drugs. Alternatively, ambulatory blood pressure monitoring (ABPM) may help to distinguish between sustained and "white coat" hypertension. The aim of treatment should be to reduce diastolic blood pressure to below 90 mm Hg. Although no firm recommendation about systolic blood pressure has been made in younger patients, it would seem prudent to reduce this to below 160 mm Hg.

The traditional approach to the drug treatment of hypertension has been "stepped care"—that is, starting treatment with a thiazide or β blocker and progressing, if necessary, to a combination of the two plus the addition of a vasodilator if needed. The introduction of calcium channel blockers and angiotensin converting enzyme (ACE) inhibitors and a resurgence in the popularity of α₁ blockers have seen a move away from this approach. Most clinicians would now favour "tailored care" to the patients' needs, which means that any of the above mentioned types of drugs could be used as first line therapy. Arguments against this approach are that the β blockers and thiazides are the only drugs that have been proved to reduce mortality and morbidity in the treatment of uncomplicated hypertension. Studies of the ability of the newer agents to prevent the complications of hypertension are, however, currently under way.

The latest guidelines of the British Hypertension Society suggest the use of β blockers or thiazides as "routine" first line drugs, but that the newer (and more expensive) drugs may be used as "alternative" first line drugs in cases where they are specifically indicated (for example, heart failure or diabetes), or where the routine agents are ineffective, cause side effects, or are specifically contraindicated.

There have been a great many clinical trials comparing different antihypertensive drugs, but there is only one reliable trial that has compared the efficacy and tolerability of all five first line drug groups—the TOMHS (Treatment Of Mild Hypertension Study)

Treatment of uncomplicated hypertension

Checklist of common or important side effects with difference classes of drug

Common side effects	Diuretic	β Blocker	Angiotensin converting enzyme inhibitor	Calcium antagonist	α₁ Blocker
Headache	−	−	−	+	−
Flushing	−	−	−	+	−
Dyspnoea	−	+	−	−	−
Lethargy	−	+	−	−	−
Impotence	+	+	−	−	−
Cough	−	−	+	−	−
Gout	+	−	−	−	−
Oedema	−	−	−	+	−
Postural hypotension	+	−	−	−	+
Cold hands and feet	−	+	−	−	−

Side effects not listed in ranking order for different classes of drugs. (From the British Hypertension Society Guidelines, in Sever (1993).)

(Neaton *et al*, 1993). The outcome of the study showed that all the major drug groups are efficacious in the treatment of mild hypertension and that the incidence of side effects and tolerability show little difference from one drug group to another.

Diuretics

Thiazide diuretics are still of value in the treatment of hypertension; they are cheap, easy to use, and can be given once daily. They are also particularly suitable for elderly and black patients. They are absorbed from the gut and excreted through the kidney.

Blood pressure is lowered by a combination of increased renal excretion of sodium and water, thereby reducing blood volume, and a direct effect on vascular smooth muscle, reducing peripheral arteriolar resistance. The dose–response curve with respect to blood pressure is flat—that is, increasing the dose beyond a certain threshold has little further antihypertensive effect. In contrast, the risks of hypokalaemia, hyperuricaemia, and hyperglycaemia continue to increase with escalating doses, so lower doses are now recommended (for example, bendrofluazide 2.5 mg or hydrochlorothiazide 25 mg once daily) than have been prescribed in the past.

Loop diuretics such as frusemide are less potent antihypertensive agents and are only indicated either when there is concomitant cardiac or renal failure, or in resistant hypertensive patients where fluid retention caused by other antihypertensive drugs may contribute to the raised blood pressure. Diuretic drugs are particularly useful in combination with β blockers and ACE inhibitors.

Thiazide diuretics

Recommended for:

Older patients

Black patients

(Loop diuretics for patients with heart failure)

Avoid in:

Maturity onset diabetics

Hyperuricaemic patients

Side effects:

Hypokalaemia

Hyperuricaemia

Hyperglycaemia

Impotence

Rashes

Blood dyscrasias

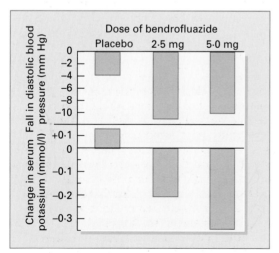

Effects of placebo and bendrofluazide, 2·5 or 5·0 mg daily, on diastolic blood pressure and serum potassium. (Adapted from Carlsen *et al*, 1990)

β Receptor antagonists

β Blockers inhibit the action of catecholamines on β adrenoreceptors. Some block both β₁ receptors (heart rate and contractility) and β₂ receptors (vascular and bronchial smooth muscle), whereas others mainly block β₁ receptors and are therefore relatively cardioselective. Used carefully they are effective and safe, and are well absorbed from the gastrointestinal tract. Some are metabolised in the liver and some excreted renally, so the dose must be reduced in patients with renal or hepatic impairment; others are excreted via either route. β Blockers are thought to lower blood pressure through a reduction in cardiac output, but they also suppress release of renin; some also have a central effect on the vasomotor centre. As with thiazide diuretics, β blockers show a flat dose–response curve for blood pressure. There is little value in increasing the dose above that recommended, although higher doses

---

β Blockers

Suitable for:

Young patients

Anxious patients

Patients with concomitant angina

Patients who have had a myocardial infarction

Non-smokers

Avoid in:

Asthma

Heart failure

Heart block

Peripheral vascular disease

Side effects:

Bronchospasm	Impaired response to hypoglycaemia
Heart failure	
Bradycardia	Hyperlipidaemia
Cold hands and feet	
Fatigue	
Vivid dreams	

There are three types of calcium channel blocker:

1 Dihydropyridines (which include nifedipine, nicardipine, and amlodipine)

2 Verapamil

3 Diltiazem

Calcium antagonists

Suitable for:

Asthmatic patients

Patients with concomitant angina

Patients wtih peripheral vascular disease

Avoid in:

Verapamil and diltiazem are contraindicated in patients with heart block	Use with care with digoxin and β blockers

Side effects:

Flushing

Headache

Ankle swelling

Constipation

Gum hyperplasia

Angiotensin converting enzyme inhibitors and β blockers are less effective in patients with low renin concentrations:

Afro-Caribbeans

Elderly people

---

may be tried in black patients because they are known to be less responsive to β blockers. The choice of β blocker depends on the other properties of these drugs:

- Lipophilic β blockers (for example, propranolol) are more likely to have side effects on the central nervous system with sleep disturbance and vivid dreams.
- Water soluble drugs (for example, atenolol) are excreted renally, have longer half lives, and can be given once daily.
- Cardioselective β blockers are less likely to affect airways resistance or raise serum cholesterol levels.
- Partial agonist activity is associated with less bradycardia and is of value in patients complaining of cold hands and feet or peripheral ischaemic symptoms.

All β blockers are contraindicated in patients with a history of wheeze or in those with either heart block on their ECG or any signs of heart failure. Clinicians should be aware of and avoid β blockers that are hidden in combination preparations, the trade name of which does not suggest the inclusion of a β blocker.

Calcium channel blockers

The calcium channel blockers are a chemically hetrogeneous group to which more drugs are being added all the time. They act through inhibition of the transfer of calcium ions across cell membranes. This transport is important for the generation of action potentials and for smooth muscle contraction. These drugs reduce blood pressure by vasodilatation. The groups of calcium channel blockers differ in their affinity for cardiac conducting tissues (slowing atrioventricular nodal conduction), cardiac muscle (reducing contractility), and vascular smooth muscle (peripheral vasodilatation). The dihydropyridines have little effect on the atrioventricular node but are potent vasodilators, and also have some mild diuretic effects. Verapamil is a useful antiarrhythmic drug with some vasodilatory action. It slows atrioventricular node conduction and reduces myocardial contractility. Diltiazem has some effect on both cardiac conduction and vascular smooth muscle. All are well absorbed from the gastrointestinal tract and undergo first pass metabolism in the liver.

Verapamil and diltiazem are contraindicated in patients with heart block and should be used with care in patients taking digoxin or the β blockers because of the additive effects on cardiac conduction and contraction. They also increase plasma concentrations of digoxin. The side effects of the dihydropyridines and diltiazem are headache and flushing which tend to improve with continued use. Ankle oedema is thought to result from a direct effect of these drugs on capillary permeability and is not responsive to diuretics. Verapamil has fewer of the side effects of the peripheral vasodilatation type, but may cause troublesome constipation.

Angiotensin converting enzyme inhibitors

The role of the renin–angiotensin–aldosterone system in the control of blood pressure has been described in the chapter on causes of hypertension. The angiotensin converting enzyme (ACE) inhibitors block this system and cause a reduction in blood pressure through a reduction in peripheral vascular resistance and, to a lesser extent, through prevention of the renal reabsorption of sodium by aldosterone. Their effects probably result through inhibition of both systemic and local tissue ACE systems. The range of available drugs is expanding, but they show little difference in their actions, except for the duration of action and route of excretion. They are all well tolerated in uncomplicated hypertension but should be used with care in elderly people, patients with renal impairment (because renal function may deteriorate), and patients taking diuretics (to avoid precipitous falls in blood pressure). Treatment should be introduced in low doses and increased gradually over the course of a few weeks.

Treatment of uncomplicated hypertension

ACE inhibitors

Recommended for:	Heart failure (but care with diuretics)
	Diabetes with proteinuria
Caution with:	• Chronic renal disease • Patients with peripheral vascular disease • Use with diuretics and non-steroidal anti-inflammatory drugs
Avoid in:	Renal artery stenosis
Side effects:	Cough
	Hypotension in volume depleted patients
	Angioneurotic oedema

The side effects of captopril were initally thought to result from its sulph-hydryl group; however, with the introduction of non-sulph-hydryl ACE inhibitors, this does not seem to be the case. The most prevalent side effect would seem to be an irritating dry cough which occurs in 10–15% of patients, and is probably more common in female non-smokers. ACE inhibitors may cause a deterioration in renal function, particularly in patients with either renal artery stenosis or pre-existing renal impairment. Rarely, these drugs may cause rashes, taste disturbance, and angio-oedema.

α Agonists

Suitable for:	Asthmatic patients
	Patients with peripheral vascular disease
	Patients with prostate symptoms/impotence
	Patients with hyperlipidaemia
Side effects:	Dry mouth
	Headaches
	Stress incontinence in women

α Receptor antagonists

Until recently, these drugs have been out of favour for the treatment of essential hypertension. With the introduction of once daily preparations (doxazosin and terazosin), however, they have experienced a resurgence in popularity. This group of drugs causes a reduction in blood pressure through antagonism of vascular α_1 adrenergic receptors, so causing arterial and venous vasodilatation. The short acting α blocker, prazosin, originally caused problems with postural hypotension. With the longer acting drugs, however, this is less of a problem. Theoretically, there are no absolute contraindications to this group of drugs. They may cause dizziness and postural hypotension, and symptoms associated with vasodilatation. A further potential benefit is that α blockers have a modest lipid lowering effect.

Angiotensin receptor antagonists

In 1995 a new class of drugs, the angiotensin (AT-1) receptor antagonists were introduced. These drugs effectively block the renin system at the level of the receptor and, therefore, do not have other effects on the bradykinin system. Perhaps as a result, this class of drug does not cause cough (unlike the ACE inhibitors). It appears that they therefore have the advantages of ACE inhibitors but none of the disadvantages, although clinical experince to date is insufficient for them to be recommended as first line therapy except possibly in patients where ACE inhibition is considered necessary but is not feasible because of cough. The first AT-1 receptor antagonist was Losartan, which is given in a starting dose of 50 mg daily.

Combination therapy

Good combinations

β Blocker plus thiazide

β Blocker plus calcium blocker

Angiotensin converting enzyme inhibitor plus diuretic

β Blocker plus α blocker

If a particular antihypertensive drug is proving ineffective, then the addition of a second drug may be the next appropriate step. As an alternative, a switch to a drug from a different group may be appropriate. Either of these steps is probably preferable to increasing the dose of the original drug to its maximum, because many side effects are dose related; as a consequence escalation of the dose may have little extra effect but produce unwanted side effects.

Bad combinations

β Blocker plus verapamil—dangerous

β Blocker plus angiotensin converting enzyme inhibitor

Calcium blocker plus thiazide

In choosing which drugs to use in combination, it is important to appreciate their modes of action and to choose a combination of drugs that complement each other. For example, the addition of a diuretic to a β blocker or ACE inhibitor is a logical step. Diuretics exert their effect on blood pressure by a reduction in the circulating volume, which is partially offset by an increase in plasma renin activity. If the renin–angiotensin sysem is subsequently blocked, this will produce a synergistic antihypertensive effect. In contrast, the combination of diuretics and calcium channel blockers is not a logical one and, in practice, produces little extra reduction in blood pressure.

Resistant hypertension

Resistant hypertension
1 Are tablets being taken?
2 Are side effects preventing adherence?
3 Check again for underlying cause

If the diastolic blood pressure is still over 100 mm Hg after triple drug treatment, consideration should be given to whether the patient is actually complying with medication. It is also worthwhile to double check that there is no underlying renal or adrenal cause for the hypertension. These patients are probably best referred to specialist hospital clinics. When essential hypertension is genuinely resistant to treatment, the substitution of frusemide for the thiazide diuretic may reduce the blood pressure.

Another approach is to use minoxidil which has a direct effect on arterioles by causing vasodilatation, although it does not dilate veins. Side effects are common so this drug is reserved for patients with genuinely severe and resistant hypertension. Fluid retention and tachycardia mean that minoxidil must be used together with a loop diuretic and a β blocker. Hypertrichosis occurs after about three weeks of treatment; it is reversible but may be cosmetically unacceptable to women.

Some patients require four or even five different antihypertensive drugs to control their blood pressure. Under these circumstances, long acting, once daily drugs are preferable.

Other drugs

Other drugs
Hydralazine
Methyldopa
Adrenergic neuron blockers, eg, bethanidine, guanethidine
Reserpine

Other drugs have been used in the past for the treatment of hypertension, although, apart from those mentioned above, few are currently used in routine practice. Hydralazine may be used for resistant heart failure in combination with nitrates, although its use for essential hypertension is much less widespread. Methyldopa has been superseded by the newer antihypertensive drugs and its use is now reserved for hypertension in pregnancy. The adrenergic neuron blockers, guanethidine and bethanidine, are no longer necessary. Reserpine is, however, still in use in some countries. In high doses, it causes depression, but is reasonably well tolerated as a first line drug in the lowest possible dose.

Further reading

Carlsen JE, Køber L, Torp-Pedersen C, Johansen, P. Relation between dose of bendrofluazide, antihypertensive effects and adverse biochemical effects. *BMJ* 1990;**300**:975–8.

Grimley Evans J, Rose G. Hypertension. *Br Med Bull* 1971;**23**:37.

Intersalt Cooperative Research Group. Intersalt: an international study of electrolyte excretion and blood pressure. Results for 24 hour urinary sodium and potassium excretion. *BMJ* 1988;**297**:19–28.

MacGregor GA, Markandu ND, Sagnella GA, Singer DRJ, Cappuccio FP. Double-blind study of three sodium intakes and long-term effect of sodium restriction in essential hypertension. *Lancet* 1989;**ii**:1244.

Neaton JD, Grim RH, Prineas RJ *et al*. Treatment of mild hypertension study: final results. *JAMA* 1993;**270**:713.

Nelson L, Jennings GL, Esler MD, Korner PJ. Effect of changing levels of physical activity on blood pressure and haemodynamics in essential hypertension. *Lancet* 1986;**ii**:473–6.

Potter JF, Beevers DG. Pressor effect of alcohol in hypertension. *Lancet* 1984;**i**:119–22.

Sever PS, Beevers G, Bulpitt C, Lever A, Ramsay L, Reid J, Swales J. Management of guidelines in essential hypotension: report of the second working party of the British Hypertension Society. *BMJ* 1993;**306**:983–7.

Staessen J, Fagard R, Amery A. Body weight and blood pressure. *J Hum Hypertens* 1989;**2**:209–18.

HYPERTENSION IN SPECIAL CASES

Factors that affect blood pressure management

Ethnic groups
Malignant hypertension
Hypertension after a stroke
Left ventricular hypertophy
Ischaemic heart disease
Heart failure
Peripheral vascular disease
Renal disease
Diabetes mellitus
Hyperlipidaemia
Connective disease tissue

The treatment of hypertension has now moved away from the concept of a rigid stepped care approach towards a view of tailoring treatment to the patient's individual needs. This chapter looks at the management of hypertension in particular groups of patients, especially those with pre-existing cardiovascular damage and those with other important concomitant medical conditions that influence the choice of treatment.

Ethnic groups

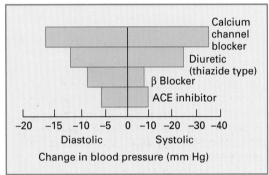

Antihypertensive drug response in black patients. (Reproduced, with permission, from Dallas Hall, 1990)

Ethnic differences and treatment

Ethnic group	
Black	High incidence of stroke
	Respond poorly to β blockers and ACE inhibitors
	More sensitive to salt
Asian	High risk of coronary heart disease
	High risk of diabetes mellitus

It is now well documented that black people have different responses to antihypertensive medication from white and Asian people, and it is thought that this is related to their low plasma renin and angiotensin levels. It has also been shown that there is a higher incidence of strokes in black hypertensive individuals so it is vital to achieve good blood pressure control. Black people are known to respond poorly to β blockers and angiotensin converting enzyme (ACE) inhibitors, although treatment with the thiazide diuretics and calcium channel blockers is effective. It has been shown, however, that the combination of diuretic therapy and ACE inhibitors is as effective in black as in white people. There is some evidence that black patients are more sensitive to salt than white patients, and advice on salt restriction is particularly important.

Hypertensive patients of Asian origin are at very high risk of coronary heart disease and diabetes mellitus. The thiazide diuretics which can worsen glucose intolerance should therefore be used with caution.

Malignant hypertension

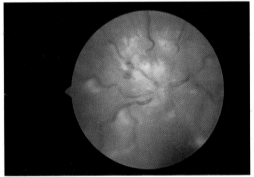

Features of hypertensive retinopathy in a patient with malignant hypertension

Malignant hypertension is diagnosed by the presence of advanced hypertensive retinopathy (haemorrhages, exudates with or without papilloedema) in the presence of a diastolic blood pressure of over 120 mm Hg. It is more common in black people and smokers. The prognosis of untreated malignant hypertension is appalling and worse than that of many neoplastic diseases. Even when treated, a high proportion of these patients develop complications such as stroke or renal failure. Again this is particularly a problem in black patients. Consequently, it is important that malignant hypertension is investigated thoroughly to exclude any cause of secondary hypertension, which is found more frequently than in non-malignant hypertension (although malignant hypertension secondary to Conn's syndrome is rare). Most patients who have malignant hypertension do not have an

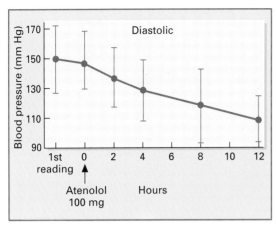

The immediate effects of treatment of malignant hypertension with 100 mg of atenolol

obvious underlying cause, although many have evidence of renal damage (for example, proteinuria). There is uncertainty about whether this results from underlying renal disease (for example, IgA nephropathy) or arteriolar necrosis caused by the malignant hypertension.

Treatment of malignant hypertension should be prompt, although it is now believed to be unnecessary and indeed unwise to treat these patients with parenteral antihypertensive medication. Precipitous falls in blood pressure from greatly raised levels may be dangerous and could lead to the development of acute stroke. Perhaps the only indications for parenteral hypertensive drugs are hypertensive encephalopathy where the patient may be unconscious or gross left ventricular failure resulting from very severe hypertension. In such cases nitroprusside or labetalol infusions may be necessary.

We suggest that blood pressure in malignant hypertension should ideally be brought down to normal over the course of a week or so. This can be achieved using a slow release preparation of nifedipine. Atenolol may be used in small doses, increasing if necessary, provided that there is no suggestion that the patient has a phaeochromocytoma. β Blockade without an α blocker may give rise to a hypertensive crisis under these circumstances. ACE inhibitors should probably not be used unless renal artery stenosis has been excluded.

Hypertension following a stroke

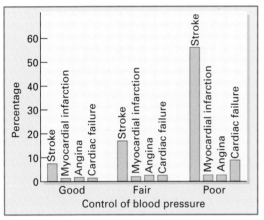

Frequency of vascular events in treated hypertensive patients following a stroke

Immediately after a stroke, there is a breakdown of cerebral autoregulation; as a result rapid falls in blood pressure can cause a reduction in cerebral perfusion and an extension of the stroke. Antihypertensive therapy is best withheld until the patient is fully ambulant. There is reliable evidence that the long term treatment of moderate to severe hypertension is associated with a reduction in incidence of subsequent strokes. The situation in mild hypertension is less clear, although most clinicians would prescribe antihypertensive drugs. If it can be proved (by CT scanning) that the stroke was the result of a cerebral infarct, then low dose aspirin is mandatory.

Left ventricular hypertrophy

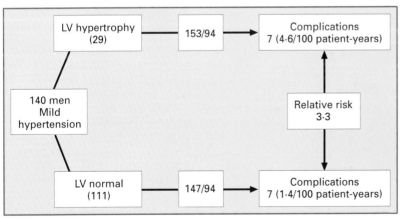

Prognostic significance of LVH on echocardiography in hypertensive patients. (From Casale et al, 1986)

The presence of left ventricular hypertrophy (LVH) is evidence of end organ damage. Left ventricular hypertrophy is an independent risk factor for cardiovascular mortality and where present, for a given level of blood pressure, the mortality is three to four times higher. It has been shown with all the drugs in current use as first line therapy that there is a reduction in left ventricular hypertrophy associated with a reduction in blood pressure.

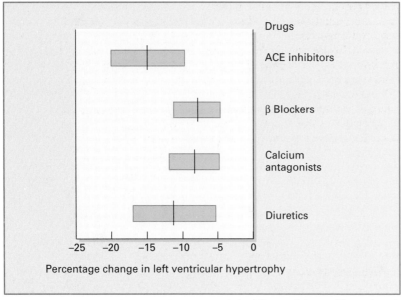

Percentage change in left ventricular mass and the effects of drugs. (Reproduced, with permission, from Dahlöf *et al*, 1992)

Two recent meta-analyses have, however, suggested that the ACE inhibitors are more effective than other drugs at reducing LVH. It is believed that this may be because angiotensin II has a growth promoting effect on cardiac muscle, mediated by tissue renin–angiotensin systems. Prospective studies are needed to show whether the reduction in left ventricular hypertrophy leads to a reduction in cardiovascular mortality and morbidity.

Ischaemic heart disease

Both angina and myocardial infarction are common in patients with hypertension. Anginal chest pain may result from coronary artery atheroma although at times it can result from relative ischaemia when left ventricular hypertrophy is not accompanied by an increase in the coronary blood supply. Many patients with angina and hypertension have normal coronary arteries on angiography. Effective management of hypertension may improve a patient's anginal symptoms regardless of the drugs used. However, the drugs of choice are those with antianginal properties; the β blockers and the dihydropyridine calcium channel blockers can be used in combination if necessary. The combination of a β blocker with verapamil is contraindicted because it can result in heart block or cardiac failure. Caution is also required when using diltiazem with a β blocker.

Following a myocardial infarction, all patients should receive aspirin and a β blocker, unless these drugs are contraindicated, because they have been shown to reduce the reinfarction rate. One study has shown some benefit in using verapamil following myocardial infarction if β blockers are contraindicated, and there is also speculation that diltiazem may be beneficial following non-q wave infarctions. Dihydropyridines (for example, nifedipine) should be avoided as one study has suggested that nifedipine may increase the risk of reinfarction.

> **Hypertensive patients after myocardial infarction**
>
> 1 If blood pressure falls—outcome poor
> 2 Other risk factors often present (smoking, hyperlipidaemia, diabetes)
> 3 Drugs that reduce the rate of reinfarction:
>   - Aspirin
>   - β Blockers
>   - Verapamil or diltiazem—one study of each only
>   - ACE inhibitors—for patients with LV impairment
> 4 Care needed because of:
>   - Low blood pressure
>   - Heart failure

There is increasing evidence that the ACE inhibitors are of value in patients following a myocardial infarction, particularly if there is evidence of compromised left ventricular function. In addition, reinfarction rates are reduced. Great care is necesary, however, to avoid excessive falls in blood pressure, particularly if diuretic therapy is being prescribed as well.

It is important to remember that there is a higher incidence of silent ischaemia or myocardial infarction in hypertensive patients. Also in the acute stages of myocardial infarction, blood pressure may have fallen so that the diagnosis of hypertension could be missed and only become apparent at subsequent clinic visits. In addition, hypertensive patients on thiazide diuretics admitted with myocardial infarction should have their potassium concentrations checked because they may have hypokalaemia which can exacerbate the tendency to arrhythmias and sudden death.

Heart failure

Hypertensive patients may develop heart failure as a result of either coronary heart disease or, occasionally, severe hypertension alone. Obviously, other forms of heart disease can occur and, in hypertensive patients, alcohol excess could provide a common aetiology. The use of

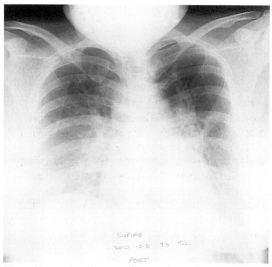

Chest X-ray showing cardiomegaly and pulmonary oedema.

Peripheral vascular disease

> Patients with peripheral vascular disease may have undiagnosed renal artery stenosis.

Renal disease

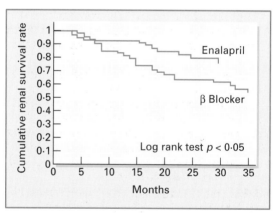

ACE inhibitors in non-diabetic renal failure. (From Hannedouche *et al*, 1994)

Drugs in renal disease

ACE inhibitors	• Care when used in conjunction with diuretic therapy • Small doses initially
β Blockers	Small doses initially
Calcium channel blockers	Relatively safe in patients with renal failure
Loop diuretics	Useful in cases of sodium and water retention

β blockers or verapamil for hypertension in patients with heart failure is contraindicated and caution should be used with diltiazem. The accepted treatment for heart failure with diuretics and ACE inhibitors could well bring the patient's blood pressure under control. The ACE inhibitors have been proved to prolong life in patients with heart failure, so they are probably the drugs of choice for patients with heart failure and hypertension. A similar although smaller benefit is also seen using a combination of hydralazine and nitrates; however, this combination is not commonly used unless ACE inhibitors are contraindicated or cause side effects.

A strong association exists between peripheral vascular disease and hypertension. Although control of blood pressure is important in these patients, caution needs to be exercised with some drugs, particularly β blockers which may worsen symptoms in patients with claudication. In addition, the presence of peripheral vascular disease may increase the likelihood of an undiagnosed atheromatous renal artery stenosis, with the consequence that the use of ACE inhibitors needs careful monitoring. Calcium channel blockers are probably the drug of choice because they are relatively safe in this condition and, in fact, they may improve the symptoms of claudication.

Renal impairment occurs with increased frequency in patients with hypertension as either a cause or an effect of the raised blood pressure. Regardless of the cause of renal impairment, hypertension has considerable influence over its progression, with good blood pressure control slowing the deterioration in renal function. In particular, ACE inhibitors have been shown to reduce microproteinuria and macroproteinuria, and there is some evidence to suggest that they preserve renal function. However, they may also precipitate a deterioration in renal function in patients with renal artery stenosis. Caution is also needed in patients with renal failure who are receiving diuretic therapy because, if they become dehydrated, the ACE inhibitors may precipitate large falls in blood pressure.

Any drugs that are excreted by the kidney (in particular, ACE inhibitors and β blockers) need to be given initially in small doses. Calcium channel blockers are effective and relatively safe in patients with renal failure, and loop diuretics may be useful, particularly if there is sodium or water retention; they may, however, need to be given in high doses.

In patients with end stage renal failure, hypertension is almost universal, but often easily controlled with dialysis. In patients who are anuric, salt and water restriction between dialyses may maintain blood pressure control, although in some drug therapy is still needed. Patients with end stage renal failure are usually anaemic, and this can be corrected by treatment with erythropoietin. However, this treatment is associated with a rise in blood pressure, the mechanisms of which are as yet unclear.

Patients with end stage renal failure, and those on dialysis or following transplantation, have a particularly high incidence of atheromatous vascular disease, heart attacks, and strokes.

Renal transplantation may obviate the need for dialysis but a high proportion of transplant recipients develop hypertension. This is more common in patients who have received kidneys from hypertensive donors. Post-transplant hypertension in the early phase may be related to acute rejection or acute tubular necrosis which follows the ischaemic period. There may be a component of fluid overload if the patient was under-dialysed before the operation, and the use of corticosteroids as immunosuppressive agents can exacerbate this. In the long term, the use of cyclosporin A may also cause hypertension, although the exact mechanisms for this are not clear.

Hypertension can develop in response to renin secretion from the patient's own atrophic kidneys, or atheromatous renal artery stenosis may affect the blood supply to the transplanted kidney; occasionally, stenosis can also occur at the surgical anastomosis. Whatever happens, adequate blood pressure control is required to preserve functioning of the transplanted kidney.

Diabetes mellitus

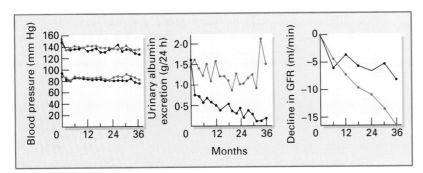

Renal protective effect of enalapril in diabetic nephropathy. (●) Enalapril; (●) metoprolol; number of patients=40. (From Björck et al, 1992)

Hypertension and diabetes commonly occur together; as they are both associated with hyperlipidaemia, this means that many patients will have three cardiovascular risk factors even if they do not smoke. All these factors should be addressed aggressively because the synergistic effects put the patient at great risk.

The aetiology of hypertension in diabetes is much debated. In insulin dependent diabetes, it is believed to result mainly from diabetic renal disease with activation of the renin–angiotensin system. In non-insulin dependent diabetes, the situation is less clear, although there seems to be volume expansion with sodium retention which may be related to hyperinsulinaemia.

Antihypertensive drugs and diabetes

α Blockers	Benefical effect on plasma lipids?
β Blockers ACE inhibitors	Safe if used carefully
Thiazide diuretics	Can worsen insulin resistance
Calcium channel blockers	Generally safe

The treatment of hypertension in diabetic patients needs to take into consideration the effects of antihypertensive drugs on glucose and lipid metabolism. α blockers are safe in this respect and may even have a beneficial effect on plasma lipids. Calcium channel blockers and ACE inhibitors are neutral and also safe when used carefully. Thiazide diuretics may worsen insulin resistance and should be used with caution in non-insulin dependent diabetic patients, although they can be used in insulin dependent patients when their effects on glucose tolerance can easily be offset by a small increase in insulin dosage. The β blockers are generally safe but some produce a lack of awareness of hypoglycaemic symptoms and should be used with caution.

There has recently been an increasing interest in the effects of ACE inhibitors on macroproteinuria or microproteinuria in diabetic patients. Proteinuria on Dipstix testing is associated with a poor prognosis; this also appears to be the case for microproteinuria (urine albumin between 20 and 200 mg/24 hours) which can be detected before Dipstix testing becomes positive. Several studies have now shown that ACE inhibitors can cause a significant reduction in urinary albumin excretion and that they may produce a slowing in the rate of deterioration of renal function. This effect seems to be independent of blood pressure control because the β blockers and the calcium channel blockers appear to have smaller effects on microproteinuria than the ACE inhibitors.

Hyperlipidaemia

The effects of antihypertensive drugs on serum lipid concentrations

	Thiazides	β Blockers		α Blockers	ACE inhibitors	Calcium blockers
		With ISA	No ISA			
Cholesterol	↑	0	↑	↓	0	0
High density lipoprotein	↓	0	↓	↑	0	0

ISA, intrinsic sympathomimetic activity.

Hyperlipidaemia when present in combination with hypertension confers a greatly increased cardiovascular risk. Fifty per cent of hypertensive patients have hyperlipidaemia, and the risk is particularly increased with higher plasma cholesterol concentrations and low HDL levels. Treatment of hyperlipidaemia should be with stringent dietetic advice; failing this, lipid lowering drugs may have to be used. Antihypertensive drugs shculd be selected on the basis of their effects on serum lipids. Thiazides and β blockers may have adverse effects on lipid profiles whereas α blockers may be beneficial. Calcium channel blockers and ACE inhibitors are lipid neutral.

Priorities and action limits for lipid lowering drug therapy in diet resistant subjects (guidelines of the British Hyperlipidaemia Association)

Priority	Subject category	Total cholesterol (mmol/l)
First	Patients with existing CHD, or post-CABG, angioplasty or cardiac transplant	>5·2
Second	Patients with multiple risk factors or genetically determined hyperlipidaemia, eg, FH	>6·5
Third	Males with asymptomatic hypercholesterolaemia	>7·8
Fourth	Postmenopausal females with asymptomatic hypercholesterolaemia	>7·8 and HDL ratio <0·2

CHD, coronary heart disease; CABG, coronary arterial bypass graft; FH, familial hypercholesterolaemia.
From Betteridge *et al*, 1993.

There is some debate about the value of lipid lowering manoeuvres in otherwise fit people. In our view, hypertensive patients who have hyperlipidaemia must be considered at high risk of heart attack, so an active lipid lowering strategy is necessary. It should be remembered, however, that plasma cholesterol concentrations do not appear to predict cardiovascular disease in patients aged 60 years or more. In such patients, lipid lowering drugs cannot be recommended unless the plasma cholesterol concentrations are consistently over 10 mmol/l.

Connective tissue diseases

The most suitable drugs for patients with connective tissue diseases

Calcium channel blockers
ACE inhibitors
α Blockers

Hypertensive patients with proteinuria should be investigated to exclude connective tissue disease

Rheumatoid arthritis, systemic lupus erythematosus, polyarteritis nodosa, and the other connective tissue disorders are all associated with renal damage and hypertension, which may be worsened through use of non-steroidal anti-inflammatory drugs, corticosteroids, and gold therapy. These treatments can raise blood pressure even further or interfere with the action of antihypertensive drugs. Overall, the most suitable drugs seem to be calcium channel blockers and ACE inhibitors, with some studies suggesting that the ACE inhibitors may protect the kidney in patients with scleroderma.

Hypertension and anaesthesia

In patients with mild hypertension many elective operations are needlessly cancelled

β Blockers may impair reflex tachycardia following blood loss and make this more difficult to diagnose.

ACE inhibitors may cause profound hypotension in patients who are volume depleted.

The problems associated with hypertension and anaesthesia can be divided into those relating to the evaluation of the blood pressure itself and those relating to the use of antihypertensive agents.

Patients who have mild symptomless hypertension, and who are otherwise fit, are at no particular risk in the perioperative period. Many non-urgent operations are postponed unnecessarily. In particular, many patients may be considerd to be hypertensive when, in fact, thay are exhibiting "white coat" hypertension associated with anxiety caused by admission to hospital. In contrast, patients who have sustained severe hypertension are at risk of perioperative arrhythmias or myocardial infarctions. In these patients elective surgery should be postponed until they have been fully assessed and their blood pressure controlled.

Anaesthesia and surgery can exacerbate problems in those patients taking particular antihypertensive medication—for example, the β blockers may block the compensatory rise in heart rate associated with fluid loss and the ACE inhibitors may block the response of the renin–angiotensin system, with the result that patients taking these drugs are prone to hypotension following blood loss. However, β blockers should not be stopped in the perioperative period, particularly in patients with coronary artery disease, because this may provoke myocardial ischaemia. The important point in the management of these patients is for the anaesthetist to be aware that the patient is taking these drugs.

In those cases where antihypertensive drugs have to be stopped because the patient cannot take them, they should be started again as soon as possible. Parenteral control of hypertension is, however, seldom indicated because patients are usually resting in bed and receiving opioid analgesia which may, in fact, reduce blood pressure.

Hypertension in children

All children with blood pressures which exceed 140/90 mm Hg should be referred to a paediatrician.

Hypertension is an uncommon problem in children and, where present, it is almost invariably the result of underlying causes. In particular, there may be renal or arteritic diseases.

Blood pressures rise sharply as children mature and those children who have higher blood pressures to start with tend to show a faster rise with advancing age. This is a particular problem in obese children. It is probable that the origins of adult essential hypertension are to be found in childhood or even infancy.

At the present state of knowledge, it is not considered justifiable to attempt to screen for hypertension in all children. However, children who have any evidence of systemic illness should have their blood pressure measured.

Under the age of three years, blood pressure measurement can only be achieved with Doppler flow equipment and, of course, at all ages, the appropriate size cuff must be employed.

Further reading

Betteridge J, Dodson PM, Durrington PN et al. Management of hyperlipidaemia: guidelines of the British Hyperlipidaemia Association. *Postgrad Med J* 1993;**69**:359.

Björck S, Mulec H, Johnsen SA, Nordén G, Aurell M. Renal protective effect of enalapril in diabetic nephropathy. *BMJ* 1992;**304**:339–43.

Casale PN, Devereux RB, Milner M et al. Value of echocardiographic measurement of left ventricular mass in predicting cardiovascular morbid events in hypertensive men. *Ann Intern Med* 1986;**105**:173–8.

Dallas Hall W. Pathophysiology of hypertension in blacks. *Am J Hypertension* 1990;**3**:366S–71S.

Dåhlof B, Pennert K, Hansson L. Reversal of left ventricular hypertrophy in hypertensive patients. A metaanalysis of 109 treatment days. *Am J Hypertension* 1992;**5**:95–110.

Hannedouche T, Landais P, Goldfarb B et al. Randomised controlled trial of enalapril and beta-blockers in non-diabetic chronic renal failure. *BMJ* 1994;**309**:833.

HYPERTENSION IN PREGNANCY

In the United Kingdom, hypertension in pregnancy is the most common cause of maternal death with a risk of around 10 per million pregnancies and it is also the most common cause of fetal and neonatal death. Unfortunately, it is still relatively poorly understood and there have been few clinical trials assessing its management. This chapter looks at different types of hypertension in pregnancy, possible mechanisms by which pregnancy induced hypertension arises, and the value of drug treatment.

Classification of hypertension in pregnancy

It is important to understand the different types of hypertension in pregnancy not least because their prognoses differ widely.

> **Classification of hypertension in pregnancy**
>
> 1 Pre-existing hypertension
>   - Essential hypertension
>   - Secondary hypertension
> 2 Pregnancy induced hypertension
> 3 Pre-eclampsia, which may lead to eclampsia

Pre-existing hypertension

Probably the most benign category is pre-existing mild essential hypertension which, of course, becomes more common with advancing maternal age. In these patients, blood pressure follows the normal pattern in pregnancy in that it may fall during the first trimester and then rise again later in the pregnancy. Of course, if blood pressures before pregnancy have not been measured, it is difficult to distinguish this from other forms of hypertension. Secondary hypertension in pregnancy may be caused by renal diseases as well as the other conditions mentioned in previous chapters. The most frequently described of these is phaeochromocytoma, which may be associated with maternal or fetal death.

Pregnancy induced hypertension

Pregnancy induced hypertension occurs in a group of patients who have normal blood pressures before and after pregnancy but whose blood pressure rises during the third trimester without the development of pre-eclampsia. This syndrome is common, occurring in up to 25% of first pregnancies although it is less common in subsequent pregnancies. It usually carries a good prognosis.

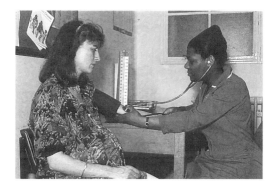

Taking blood pressure of a pregnant woman

Pre-eclampsia

The diagnosis of pre-eclampsia depends on the presence of proteinuria accompanied by a rise in blood pressure to over 140/90 mm Hg in the second half of pregnancy. Pre-eclampsia is less common than pregnancy induced hypertension, occurring in about 5% of first pregnancies. The prevalence falls in subsequent pregnancies by the same father, but pregnancies by different fathers are said to have the same rate as in primigravidae. The prognosis of pre-eclampsia is much more sinister than the other hypertensive pregnancy syndromes.

Eclampsia

Full blown eclampsia is an obstetric emergency with a very high risk to the mother and fetus. In addition to hypertension and proteinuria, there is often gross oedema, and the more serious complications include cerebral oedema with convulsions, renal failure, pulmonary oedema, and disseminated intravascular coagulation. Fortunately, this condition is rare in developed countries, occurring in about 1 in 500 pregnancies.

Aetiology of pre-clampsia

Features of pre-eclampsia

Clinical

(1) Proteinuria
(2) Hypertension
(3) Oedema (mild oedema occurs in normal pregnancies)
(4) Rapid weight gain

Investigations

(1) Thrombocytopenia
(2) Hyperuricaemia
(3) Intrauterine growth retardation on ultrasonography
(4) Fall in fetal heart rate

High risk groups

Primigravidae
Teenage mothers
History of raised blood pressure
Diabetic mothers
Twin pregnancies
Low social class
Rhesus isoimmunisation
Previous oral contraceptive hypertension (weak association)

Pre-eclampsia has several risk factors in common with hypertension in non-obstetric practice. For example, it seems to be more common in those with a family history of pre-eclampsia, in obese mothers, in diabetic patients, and in those of low socioeconomic status. There is an increasing incidence of pre-eclampsia with advancing maternal age but, paradoxically, there is also high incidence in young teenage mothers.

Other risk factors are related to the patient's obstetric history. Pre-eclampsia is more common in first pregnancies or subsequent pregnancies by different fathers. Although the risk of pre-eclampsia in mothers who have previously had it is increased, it is still relatively low. In addition, pre-eclampsia is associated with multiple pregnancies, hydaditiform mole, and rhesus isoimmunisation.

It is now becoming clear that the origins of pre-eclampsia lie in abnormalities of implantation of the placenta in the first trimester. Failure of the development of the placental blood vessels leads to placental and fetal ischaemia in severe cases, and eventually to placental infarctions. The fetus may suffer intrauterine growth retardation as it becomes hypoxic and ischaemic; occasionally it dies. It is unclear how this disease progresses to produce the syndrome of hypertension and proteinuria. The circulating renin–angiotensin system is certainly less activated than in normal pregnancies and, although there are disturbances of other vasoactive systems such as the kallikrein–kinin system and endothelin, the significance of these is not fully understood.

Management of hypertension in pregnancy

Hazards of hypertension in pregnancy

To the mother:
Renal failure
Stroke
Eclamptic fits
Hepatic failure
Retinal detachment
Papilloedema
Irritability

To the baby:
Placental insufficiency
Placental infarctions
Intrauterine growth retardation
Intrauterine death

The care of obstetric patients should probably start before they become pregnant. This entails monitoring the blood pressures of the young female population so that their baseline blood pressures are documented. Many women may be found to be mildly hypertensive, but treatment may not be required because these patients have low absolute risk of developing cardiovascular complications. However, if treatment is instigated, ideally it should be with a drug that can be used safely in women who become pregnant. As in a non-pregnant state, special efforts should be made to avoid unnecessary treatment where the blood pressure is temporarily raised due to anxiety, perhaps using ambulatory monitoring to avoid undue delay in diagnosis.

Mild hypertension in pregnancy with pressures below 150/100 mm Hg, particularly if detected in the first 20 weeks of gestation, should usually not be treated with drugs. This is because the raised blood pressure is probably caused by mild essential hypertension, and there is evidence to suggest that these women have no increase in perinatal mortality. These patients should, however, undergo basic investigation. If hypertension is more severe, then antihypertensive medication should be started, occasionally after admission to hospital for assessment. The development of proteinuria in association with hypertension in the second half of pregnancy implies a diagnosis of pre-eclampsia. These women should always be admitted to hospital for full assessment and control of their blood pressure. If pre-eclampsia develops near the end of the pregnancy, the optimum treatment is delivery of the baby while maintaining good blood pressure control.

Blood pressure reduction in pregnancy

Non-pharmacological manoeuvres to reduce blood pressure in pregnancy have not been extensively addressed. Strict bed rest is not indicated and may be harmful, but reduced physical activity may be appropriate.

Drug treatment when indicated must take into consideration any potential effects of antihypertensive drugs on the fetus. Angiotensin converting enzyme inhibitors are absolutely contraindicated in pregnancy because they have been associated with congenital abnormalities, growth retardation, intrauterine death, and fetal anuria. The calcium channel blocker, nifedipine, has been used safely in severe resistant hypertension. However, the calcium channel blockers should not be used for mild hypertension because there is little information available about their use. The α blockers are probably safe but the newer ones, such as doxazosin, have yet to undergo formal testing.

Until recently, β blockers and methyldopa have formed the mainstay of treatment. However, information is now available to suggest that atenolol may be associated with reduced fetal blood flow and smaller babies. It is thought that this is because of its lack of intrinsic sympathomimetic activity. The other β blockers, such as oxprenolol and pindolol, may be safer; the combined α and β blocker, labetalol, has been used extensively and shown not to be associated with growth retardation. Methyldopa is the drug of choice in asthmatic mothers, although it has recently moved out of favour as first line treatment because it can cause sedation and lethargy and possibly postnatal depression.

Diuretics are generally not used to treat hypertension in pregnancy. In particular, the thiazides, through a reduction in circulating volume, may cause an impairment of uteroplacental blood flow.

In the emergency management of hypertension in mothers with eclampsia, intravenous and intramuscular drugs may be required such as hydralazine or labetalol, together with anticonvulsants. These patients should be admitted to well equipped and staffed obstetric units with adequate facilities for neonatal care.

Aspirin

There is evidence that low dose aspirin is beneficial in high risk pregnancies, and this is usually given until about three weeks before a planned delivery. There is as yet no information on its use in mothers with hypertension. It is probably best to reserve it for use in those cases where there has been a previous history of intrauterine death, still birth, or growth retardation.

Drug treatments

Contraindicated
ACE inhibitors
Calcium channel blockers (except in severe hypertension)
Thiazides

Suitable
α Blockers
β Blockers, eg, oxprenolol, pindolol
Methyldopa—particularly in asthmatic mothers
Nifedipine in severe cases
Aspirin—in high risk mothers

Emergency
Intravenous and intramuscular drugs, eg, hydralazine, labetalol
Anticonvulsants

Conclusion

The decision to give antihypertensive treatment should not be taken lightly

There has, over the past 10 years, been an increasing tendency to withhold drug therapy in mothers with blood pressures below 150/100 mm Hg. The decision to give drugs to pregnant women should probably only be made by highly qualified obstetricians or physicians with special experience of managing hypertension in pregnancy.

Further reading
National High Blood Pressure Education Program Working Group. Report on High Blood Pressure in Pregnancy. *Am J Obstet Gynecol* 1986;**163**:1689–712.

HYPERTENSION IN PRIMARY CARE

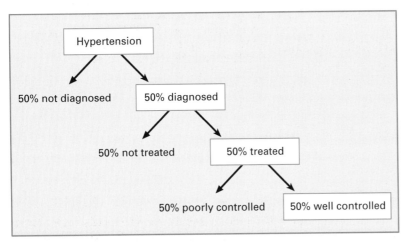

The rule of halves

There is firm evidence that the accurate detection, assessment, and treatment of hypertensive patients is a well validated medical intervention because it leads to a significant reduction in the number of strokes and heart attacks. Sadly, however, there is also evidence that a very large number of hypertensive patients are not receiving the treatment they need as a result of deficiencies in the methods of delivery of health care. The "rule of halves" (an expression first coined in the 1960s) still prevails unless special efforts are made.

As the vast majority of hypertensive patients do not (and should not) attend hospital, it is clear that the management of millions of mildly hypertensive patients can only be achieved within the context of primary health care. The systems for delivery of primary health care differ among nations but the principles remain the same everywhere.

In the United Kingdom the routine measurement of blood pressure in all people is now considered to be an integral part of good medical care. All British citizens have a named general practitioner or family doctor. Evidence that blood pressures are being measured routinely is now being demanded by health care administrators and suitable clinical audit programmes are being devised.

In addition, there has been an expansion in the number of nurse practitioners working in close collaboration with general practitioners. These nurses can, with adequate training, organise the detection, management, and follow up of most hypertensive patients.

Screening

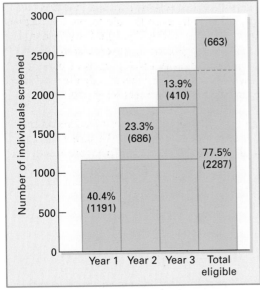

"Opportunistic screening." General practice case detection of hypertension in men aged 35–69 years: taken from records of six general practitioners. (From Barber *et al*, 1979)

As hypertension is usually an asymptomatic condition, clearly some form of screening is necessary to detect cases. Although dedicated screening units can help, these are not, in general, to be encouraged because they do not have the appropriate methods of follow up and are often organised on a "one-off" basis. The ongoing screening of symptomless patients for high blood pressure should, therefore, take place within the context of primary health care.

As between 70% and 80% of the population are likely to visit a doctor at least once in three years, it is preferable that screening should take place at the same time. This system referred to as "opportunistic screening" has been demonstrated to be effective in general practice in both a city centre and rural environment. All patients who visit their general practitioners should have their blood pressure checked if they have not attended for more than 12 months. All those whose blood pressures exceed 160/90 mm Hg should be advised that their blood pressures are not quite normal and recalled for re-examination a few weeks later. The nurse practitioner is the best member of the health care team to arrange this procedure.

Assessment

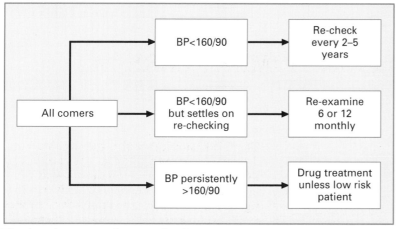

The three box system for assessing blood pressure

If, after four consultations, the systolic blood pressure still exceeds 160 mm Hg and the diastolic blood pressure 90 mm Hg, then more detailed assessment is necessary. All such patients should undergo a routine urine test, a single blood test to measure renal function and serum cholesterol concentration, and an ECG to assess left ventricular size.

The optimum method of managing these patients is that set out in the guidelines suggested by the British Hypertension Society in 1993 (Sever *et al*, 1993). Similar useful guidelines have also been produced in New Zealand and the United States.

High risk groups

High risk groups

1 People with a family history of hypertension, heart attack, or stroke
2 Patients with a previous vascular complication of hypertension
3 Patients with diabetes mellitus
4 Patients with other systemic diseases, including renal disease, polyarteritis, systemic lupus erythematosus, and peripheral vascular disease
5 Pregnant women

Certain patient groups should be sought out specifically rather than waiting for them to attend for some other reason. It is possible that special appointments should be sent to such patients. This "selective screening" might be conducted in patients who are at particular risk of developing hypertension or its vascular complications, including those shown in the box.

Medical records

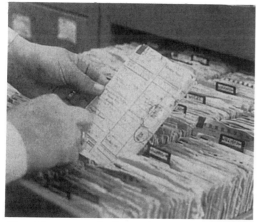

Lloyd George medical record system in general practice

If chronic diseases such as hypertension are to be managed efficiently then it is necessary to have good medical records. The increasing sophistication of computer hardware and software means that this can be achieved without difficulty. However, even the old fashioned records system still used in some health centres in the UK (the Lloyd George envelope) can be adapted for the management of hypertension. A system of flags can be introduced to identify three groups of patients: those who have never had their blood pressure measured; those who require regular monitoring; and those who are receiving drug treatment.

Computerised systems can render clinical audit very feasible so that clinicians can investigate how frequently they reach the target for the detection of hypertension and introduction of blood pressure treatment.

Specialist referral

About 10% of hypertensive patients in primary health care have underlying causes for their high blood pressure or have very severe or resistant hypertension. Most of these patients need referral to a specialist centre for detailed investigation and management.

Cardiovascular prevention in general practice

The vast majority of hyertensive patients can be managed exclusively in the primary care context. It is important, however, that primary care nurses and clinicians are kept in touch with the new information that is continuing to become available (several important papers on the treatment of hypertension have been published since 1991). It is important that public health physicians and administrators make special efforts to ensure that health care providers are up to date and are achieving the appropriate targets.

We now have reliable evidence that almost all strokes that are caused by hypertension can be prevented with accurate antihypertensive antihypertensive treatment. There is also evidence that a substantial impact can be made on the incidence of coronary heart disease. The prime responsibility for the administration of this validated health care rests in general practice, but considerable changes are necessary in the way that clinicians practise medicine (particularly for chronic diseases). It is the responsibility of general practitioners to seek out people who night have hypertension rather than waiting for them to present at a late stage of their disease, when they become clinically unwell with cardiovascular complications. General practitioners are, thus, responsible for the health of all the patients allocated to them and not just to those presenting with clinical illness.

In the United Kindom, family doctors are remunerated partly on the basis of the number of people aged 15–74 years screened from their allotted patient list. This should lead to 90% of the population having a blood pressure check within five years.

The benefits of controlling hypertension		
	Predicted (%)	Achieved (%)
Stroke prevention	35–40	38±4
CHD prevention	20–25	16±4

From Collins and MacMahon (1994).

Hypertension clinics

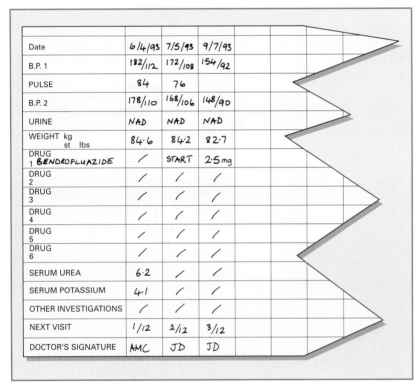

Date	6/4/93	7/5/93	9/7/93			
B.P. 1	182/112	172/108	154/92			
PULSE	84	76				
B.P. 2	178/110	168/106	148/90			
URINE	NAD	NAD	NAD			
WEIGHT kg st lbs	84·6	84·2	82·7			
DRUG 1 BENDROFLUAZIDE	/	START	2·5 mg			
DRUG 2	/	/	/			
DRUG 3	/	/	/			
DRUG 4	/	/	/			
DRUG 5	/	/	/			
DRUG 6	/	/	/			
SERUM UREA	6·2	/	/			
SERUM POTASSIUM	4·1	/	/			
OTHER INVESTIGATIONS	/	/	/			
NEXT VISIT	1/12	2/12	3/12			
DOCTOR'S SIGNATURE	AMC	JD	JD			

An example of a patient held hypertension cooperation card

Many general practitioners have established dedicated hypertension clinics to achieve efficient ongoing care of their patients. These clinics can best be run by appropriately trained and supervised nurse practitioners with well devised computerised medical records. Patient held hypertension cooperation cards are useful if hospital clinic attendance is also necessary.

Further reading

Barber JH, Beevers DG, Fife R *et al*. Blood-pressure screening and supervision in general practice. *BMJ* 1979;i:843–6.

Collins R, MacMahon S. Blood pressure, antihypertensive drug therapy and risk of stroke coronary heart disease. *Br Med Bull* 1994;50:272–98.

Sever P, Beevers G, Bulpitt C, Lever A, Ramsay L, Reid J, Swales, J. Management guidelines in essential hypertension: report of the second working party of the British Hypertension Society. *BMJ* 1993;**306**:983–7.

INDEX

Abbreviations; BP, blood pressure; CV, cardiovascular

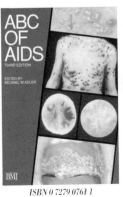
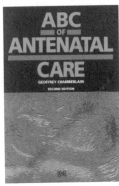
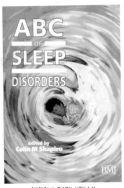
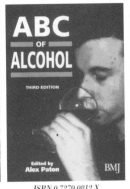
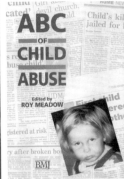
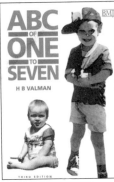
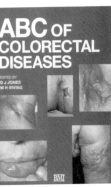
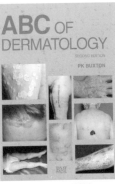
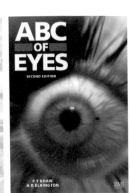
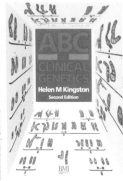
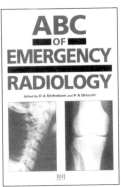
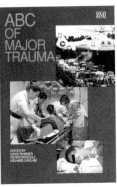
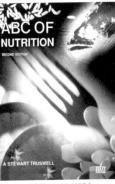
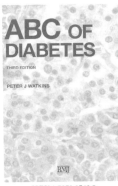
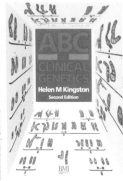
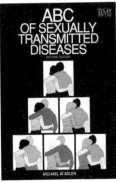
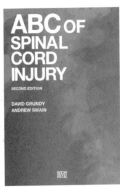
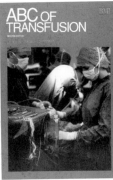
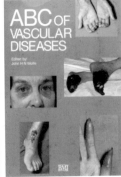
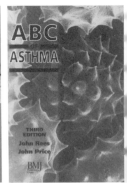
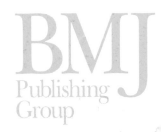